The
Prostatitis
Manual

The Prostatitis Manual

A practical guide to
management of prostatitis/
chronic pelvic pain syndrome

J CURTIS NICKEL

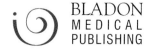
BLADON
MEDICAL
PUBLISHING

© 2002
by Bladon Medical Publishing

12 New Street, Chipping Norton,
Oxfordshire OX7 5LJ, UK

First published 2002

British Library Cataloguing in
Publication Data.

A catalogue record for this title is
available from the British Library

ISBN 1-904218-08-3

Nickel, J.C. The Prostatitis Manual

Design and production:
Design Online Ltd, Oxford

Printed by
Grafiche IGC S.R.L.,
25128 Brescia, Zona Industriale,
Via A. Grandi, 29, Italy

Distributed by
Plymbridge Distributors Ltd,
Estover Road, Plymouth
PL6 7PY, U

CONTENTS

FOREWORD   Daniel Shoskes MD   vii

INTRODUCTION   ix

CHAPTER 1
THE PROBLEM WITH PROSTATITIS   1

THE PROSTATITIS PATIENT   2
Who is the patient with prostatitis?   2
The incidence/prevalence of prostatitis   2
The costs of prostatitis   3
Quality of life of prostatitis patients   4

THE PHYSICIAN WHO TREATS PROSTATITIS   6
The frustrated physician   6
What percentage of practice is devoted to prostatitis?   6
The standard diagnostic and treatment plan   7

A HISTORY LESSON: 100 YEARS OF PROGRESS?   10
Before antibiotics   10
Prostatitis as an infectious disease   10
Perhaps prostatitis is not always an infectious disease   12
A 'best evidence-based' strategy   12
Suggested Reading   14

CHAPTER 2
ETIOLOGY OF PROSTATITIS: WHAT DO WE REALLY KNOW?   15

INFECTIOUS   16
Historical record   16
Do bacteria cause the symptoms?   17
Other micro-organisms   17
Previous history of infection   18

ANATOMIC   21

TRAUMATIC   23

IMMUNOLOGIC   24

NEUROMUSCULAR   25

INTERSTITIAL CYSTITIS   26

A MULTIFACTORIAL INTER-RELATED CASCADE:
THE FINAL PATHWAY   26

Suggested Reading   28

CHAPTER 3
EVALUATION OF THE PROSTATITIS PATIENT:
THE FIRST STEP IN MANAGEMENT   29

CLASSIFICATION SYSTEM FOR CLINICAL PRACTICE   30

CLINICAL DIAGNOSIS   33

Acute bacterial prostatitis (Category I)   33

Chronic bacterial prostatitis (Category II)   33

Chronic non-bacterial prostatitis/prostatodynia
(Category III: chronic pelvic pain syndrome)   34

A SYMPTOM ASSESSMENT TOOL   35

A SIMPLE LOWER URINARY TRACT LOCALIZATION TECHNIQUE   38

OTHER TESTS   46

Semen analysis   47

Urethral swab   47

Cytological examination of the urine   48

Prostate specific antigen   48

Cystoscopy   50

Transrectal ultrasound   50

Abdominal/pelvic ultrasound, CAT scan, MRI   51

Urodynamics   52

Suggested Reading   54

CHAPTER 4
PRACTICAL THERAPEUTIC STRATEGIES FOR THE PROSTATITIS
PATIENT: DEVELOPMENT OF A TREATMENT PLAN   55

ACUTE BACTERIAL PROSTATITIS (CATEGORY I): A SPECIAL CASE   56
Optimize urinary drainage   56
Eradicate the bacteria   56
Supportive care   57
Close follow-up   57

CHRONIC BACTERIAL PROSTATITIS (CATEGORY II)   58
Antibiotics   58
Prostate massage   60
Alpha-blockers   60
Surgery   60

CHRONIC PROSTATITIS/CHRONIC PELVIC PAIN SYNDROME
(CATEGORY III)   62
Conservative therapy   63
Antibiotics   65
Alpha-blockers   68
Anti-inflammatories   69
Hormone therapy   71
Muscle relaxants   71
Phytotherapeutic agents (plant extracts) and other supplements   72
Other medical therapies   73
Physical therapies   75
Minimally invasive therapies   76
Surgery   78

ASYMPTOMATIC INFLAMMATORY PROSTATITIS (CATEGORY IV)   79

Suggested Reading   80

CONTENTS

CHAPTER 5

PRACTICAL STRATEGIES FOR THE TREATMENT OF PATIENTS
WITH PROSTATITIS: A CLINICAL ALGORITHM   81

CATEGORY I: ACUTE BACTERIAL PROSTATITIS   82

CATEGORY II/III: CHRONIC PROSTATITIS /
CHRONIC PELVIC PAIN SYNDROME   83

The patient contract   83

The investigation   83

The patient with Category II chronic bacterial prostatitis   85

The patient with Category III chronic pelvic pain syndrome   86

CATEGORY IV: ASYMPTOMATIC INFLAMMATORY PROSTATITIS   90

Suggested Reading   92

CHAPTER 6

THE FUTURE FOR PROSTATITIS MANAGEMENT: A LIGHT AT THE
END OF THE TUNNEL   93

ETIOLOGY   94

DIAGNOSIS   94

TREATMENT   95

THE EVOLVING FIELD OF PROSTATITIS MANAGEMENT   96

Suggested Reading   96

CHAPTER 7
BIBLIOGRAPHY   97

INDEX   111

FOREWORD

Chronic prostatitis has been a backwater of clinical and basic science urology research over the past few decades. Most physicians have a vague feeling that these patients have a chronic infection even though cultures are seldom positive (if they are even performed) and many patients get no improvement despite kilograms of antibiotics over months or years. It's not as though academic researchers have given much guidance to practitioners; amazingly there are only a handful of small randomized placebo-controlled studies for therapy in chronic prostatitis, the vast majority being for documented bacterial prostatitis, which makes up fewer than 10% of those patients we see in practice.

Over the past two decades, Dr Nickel has devoted his prodigious talent and energy towards understanding this disease and testing novel therapies. Thanks to him and like-minded researchers, there is a greater understanding of the heterogeneity of the condition we now call 'chronic pelvic pain syndrome' and new rational therapeutic options which can be effective for the majority of patients. In this handbook, the first of its kind for chronic prostatitis, Dr Nickel succinctly summarizes the current understanding of the pathophysiology, evaluation and treatment options available for these patients. Particularly illuminating is the history lesson, which demonstrates in sobering detail how little progress has been made until most recently.

This guide presents a clear stepwise approach to the management of these challenging patients in clinical practice. For the student and resident it summarizes all the didactic and clinical information they need to know. For the experienced clinician, it can provide a roadmap to novel therapies to assist in the management of their most difficult patients who are refractory to conventional treatments.

Daniel Shoskes MD
Cleveland Clinic - Florida

INTRODUCTION

In 1999, I edited the Textbook of Prostatitis, an exhaustive up-to-date compendium of knowledge in the rapidly changing field of prostatitis research. This first attempt to compile the world's knowledge on the epidemiology, etiology, diagnosis, and treatment of prostatitis was written by the best known and respected international clinicians and researchers in the field. The Textbook of Prostatitis is a wonderful tool for clinicians and researchers who have a primary interest in prostatitis. However, it has become apparent that the book was too large and covered the topic too comprehensively to be of value to students learning about the condition and physicians who manage these patients. Based on this type of feedback, we could see a definite need for a clinical manual on prostatitis, one which would present the practical data and information the physician requires to effectively diagnose and treat prostatitis patients who present to their clinic. This Prostatitis Manual does just that. It distills a century of research, diagnostic approaches, and therapeutic plans into a 'best evidence-based management plan' for the diagnosis and treatment of prostatitis.

CHAPTER 1
THE PROBLEM WITH PROSTATITIS

The prostatitis syndromes have been frustrating physicians and patients for most of the last century. Recent studies have illuminated the scope of the problem, both in terms of the number of patients affected and the difficulties faced by both physicians and patients in tackling this problem. A historic overview suggests that progress has been made over the last century, but we have not yet found the cause or the cure for many of the patients suffering from prostatitis syndromes. However, new initiatives by a committed group of interested and qualified researchers, stimulated by local, government and industry funding, have resulted in more progress in this field in the last 10 years than was made in the last 100 years.

THE PROSTATITIS PATIENT

Who is the patient with prostatitis?

Most clinicians who evaluate and treat prostatitis patients would tell you that these patients are easy to identify, but difficult to diagnose and categorize. Clinicians have no problem diagnosing the patient arriving in the emergency department or their clinic with acute perineal and suprapubic pain, fever and chills and irritative and obstructive voiding symptoms. These patients with 'acute bacterial prostatitis' pose no diagnostic and therapeutic dilemma. It is the majority of the patients who present with genitourinary and pelvic pain, associated with irritative and obstructive voiding symptoms and variable sexual dysfunction, who present a challenge. The very rare patient will have a history of recurrent urinary tract infections and clinical exacerbations resolve with antibiotic therapy. Some patients present for the first time with a recent constellation of symptoms that resolve quickly with appropriate medical therapy, never to return to the clinician's office again. However, most patients have a long history of distress; waxing and waning pain, bothersome voiding symptoms, painful and difficult sexual experiences and a dismal quality of life. While it has generally been believed, and taught, that benign prostatic hyperplasia and prostate cancer are diseases of older men (true), prostatitis was a condition that generally affected younger men. Recent epidemiological data do not support that generally held belief. Prostatitis-like symptoms can occur in men of all ages, from the very young to the very old.

The incidence/prevalence of prostatitis

In the past, well-respected researchers in the field, like Thomas Stamey of Stanford University, suggested that as many as 25% of men experienced

THE PROBLEM WITH PROSTATITIS
THE PROSTATITIS PATIENT
Who is the patient with prostatitis?
The incidence/prevalence of prostatitis
The costs of prostatitis

symptoms of prostatitis sometime in their life. An extensive community-based survey of family physicians' offices in Olmsted County, a county in Minnesota near the Mayo Clinic that has become one of the most famous areas for epidemiological study in urologic diseases, noted that 11% of men had a physician diagnosis of prostatitis. A similar study conducted in Finland, based on patients' recollection of a prostatitis diagnosis, demonstrated that 14% of fit men in the Oulu district of Finland had a current or previous diagnosis of prostatitis. At any one time, it has been estimated from population-based studies in Canada, the USA, and Singapore that 2–6% of men in the community are experiencing at least mild to moderate prostatitis-like symptoms. There is absolutely no doubt that prostatitis-like symptoms and prostatitis diagnoses by physicians are extremely common.

The costs of prostatitis

Prostatitis results in a significant economic cost to both individual patients and to society itself. The impact of this condition makes it impossible for many patients to do the mental and physical activities they would like to do or accomplish goals that they have set out for themselves. Most of these patients are in the age category that has many years to contribute to the betterment of their community. Physician visits, diagnostic testing, long-term medical therapy, alternate minimally invasive therapies and surgery in some instances, are expensive. Until recently, this major cost to society was not fully appreciated. A National Institutes of Health Chronic Prostatitis Collaborative Research Network study examined the socioeconomic impact of a prostatitis diagnosis in men who had the condition for longer than 3 months. This study discovered, to no one's real surprise, that the economic costs were enormous. Extrapolations of these specific costs, based on the estimated number of patients in the USA alone, would reach hundreds of millions and perhaps even billions of dollars per year in that country alone. Economic costs associated with the time off work, disability and loss of personal productivity would significantly increase those estimated costs. Prostatitis is a major socioeconomic burden on our society.

The quality of life of prostatitis patients

The effect of this particular disease, syndrome or constellation of symptoms on a patient's quality of life can be accurately estimated and compared to other diseases for which quality of life and impact have been determined. When such comparisons are made, it becomes evident that

KEY POINTS

The Prostatitis Patient

- 11-14% of men have had a current or previous diagnosis of prostatitis

- 2-6% of men experience at least mild to moderate prostatitis-like symptoms at any particular time

- prostatitis represents a major socioeconomic burden

- the quality of life of a patient diagnosed with chronic prostatitis is dismal

THE PROBLEM WITH PROSTATITIS
THE PROSTATITIS PATIENT
The costs of prostatitis
The quality of life of prostatitis patients

the quality of life of a patient diagnosed with chronic prostatitis is dismal. It is comparable to patients who have just had an acute myocardial infarction, or suffer from unstable angina, active Crohn's disease, congestive heart failure or severe diabetes mellitus. It appears the symptoms associated with prostatitis affect both the physical and mental aspects of the patient's quality of life, but the mental health impact is more profound. Recent studies have confirmed that prostatitis patients spend a significant amount of their waking hours thinking about their condition. These studies have also confirmed that the symptoms prevent the patients from doing the normal day-to-day activities that they would like to do. Very few patients diagnosed with chronic prostatitis are happy with their quality of life. It is very evident that patients with prostatitis do not have an enviable quality of life.

Impact on
Quality of Life

Voiding
Problems

Pain & Discomfort

Sexual
Problems

The inter-related domains of pain, disturbed voiding, sexual difficulties and impact on quality of life that make up the life experience of a patient with chronic prostatitis

5

THE PHYSICIAN WHO TREATS PROSTATITIS

The frustrated physician

Who diagnoses and treats prostatitis? Patients presenting acutely with
bacterial prostatitis are usually seen by the casualty officer, emergency
room physician or primary care family physician. Although this type of
presentation is rare, these physicians are trained to recognize a lower
urinary tract infection, likely originating in the prostate gland and can
effectively make diagnostic and therapeutic decisions regarding the need
for cultures, bladder drainage and antibiotics. Depending on the medical
system in any one country, patients with chronic prostatitis-like symptoms
are seen first by a primary care family physician or a urologist. Primary
care physicians for the most part, appear frustrated by lack of specific
knowledge of appropriate diagnostic and therapeutic maneuvers. North
American surveys of primary care physicians have shown that the average
primary care physician will undertake a physical examination, usually
with a digital rectal examination (DRE), arrange for a urine culture and
then treat the patient with antibiotics. The initial antibiotics prescribed
and the duration of therapy vary widely. There appears to be no rationale
for either selection or duration of antibiotic therapy among the primary
care physician community. If patients respond to antibiotic therapy (and
many do) the patient is seldom referred on for an expert opinion. However,
in many cases the patient does not respond or the symptoms recur after
antibiotics are discontinued and the patient is subsequently referred along
to a urologist (and sometimes an infectious diseases specialist).

What percentage of practice is devoted to prostatitis

The reason for the confusion among primary care physicians as to an
appropriate diagnostic and therapeutic plan becomes obvious when one

THE PROBLEM WITH PROSTATITIS
THE PHYSICIAN WHO TREATS PROSTATITIS
The frustrated physician
What percentage of practice is devoted to prostatitis
The standard diagnostic and treatment plans

surveys the activities of the urology communities in the field. The average North American urologist sees between 100 and 150 prostatitis patients per year, one-third of them new to their practice. Since some urologists see no prostatitis patients, many urologists see more patients than this. A prostatitis diagnosis represents 8% of patients' visits to urologists; it is the most common urologic diagnosis made in men under 50 years of age and the third most common urologic diagnosis made in men over 50. Patients with prostatitis become frustrated with the medical profession and those with persistent symptoms tend to shop around for physicians who may hold the clue to ameliorating or curing their symptoms. Patients who have suffered symptoms for more than 2 years have often seen more than three urologic specialists for opinions.

The standard diagnostic and treatment plans

European, Canadian and US studies all confirm that there is no unified, accepted diagnostic or therapeutic plan for patients presenting with chronic prostatitis symptoms. Although the majority of urologists will at least perform a digital rectal examination and a simple urine culture, most do not proceed with any more specific diagnostic testing of prostatitis patients. The primary choice of therapy for urologists and prostatitis patients, regardless of culture results, is antibiotics. The antibiotics of choice are the quinolones, trimethoprim-sulfamethoxazole and trimethoprim. Urologists' rationale for these antibiotics is based on a faint recollection of the results of animal studies performed in the 1970s which suggested that these antibiotics penetrate the prostate better than other antibiotics. Alpha-blockers and anti-inflammatory agents appear to be the second and third most common treatments prescribed by urologists. Patients tend to treat themselves with many over-the-counter

The standard diagnostic and treatment plans

supplements and plant extracts. Surveys have confirmed that urologists are not happy with this management scenario. Most realize that, compared with diagnostic steps they take in other urologic diseases, their evaluation and categorization of prostatitis patients is poor. Most will also concede that empiric treatment, practiced by the majority of urologists, is ill-conceived and in many instances ineffective. The level of frustration among urologists dealing with prostatitis patients is evident. Given a choice, many urologists would decline to see these patients and many refuse to see patients again once they fail their initial prescription. Urologists have rated prostatitis as one of the most difficult and frustrating disease entities that they manage.

KEYPOINTS

The Physician Who Treats Prostatitis

- prostatitis is the most common urologic diagnosis made in men under 50

- prostatitis diagnoses represent 8% of patients' visits to urologists

- the average North American urologist sees 100-150 prostatitis patients per year

- physicians concede that empiric therapy is ill-conceived and usually ineffective

- urologists have rated prostatitis as the most difficult and frustrating condition that they manage

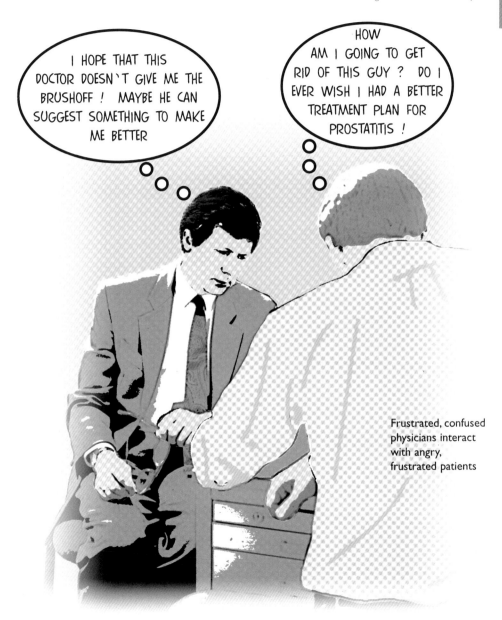

Frustrated, confused physicians interact with angry, frustrated patients

A HISTORY LESSON: 100 YEARS OF PROGRESS

Before antibiotics

The medical professions' experience with the diagnosis and treatment of prostatitis is not new. In the late 1800s the development of prostatitis symptoms was believed to be associated with repetitive perineal trauma (horseback riding or riding on hard seats in poorly suspended horse-drawn buggies) and excessive or abnormal sexual practices. In the pre-Pasteur age of microbiology and before antibiotics were introduced, a prostate infection was a major potentially fatal medical problem. Prostatic abscess, either secondary to gonococcal urethritis or bacterial prostatitis was a serious, often fatal disease and was treated primarily by surgical incision and drainage. Following the introduction of antibiotic therapy, prostate abscesses, which still occur, have become much less common and are associated with acute bacterial prostatitis and not the chronic prostatitis syndromes.

Prostatitis as an infectious disease

Following the exciting introduction by Pasteur and other microbiologists of the story on the microbial etiology of infectious diseases, urologists became enthused about the possibility that prostatitis was actually an infectious disease. Large and elaborate bacterial localization studies, involving thousands of patients, were presented and published in the 1920s and 1930s. Researchers from that era concluded that all prostatitis symptoms were secondary to bacterial pathogens, likely gram-positive organisms (usually coagulase-negative *Staphylococcus* or *Streptococcus* species). These studies became even more important following the introduction of the new antibiotics. While decades of progress in microbiological research and antibiotic therapy eliminated or improved the prognosis of patients with other infectious diseases, the same thing cannot be said for prostatitis. Later in the 1950s and 1960s questions arose as to whether or not the bacteria cultured were really causing the symptoms. Control studies of asymptomatic men showed similar microbiological profiles. Antibiotics did not appear to be a panacea and in fact in most patients did very little to ameliorate the chronic symptoms.

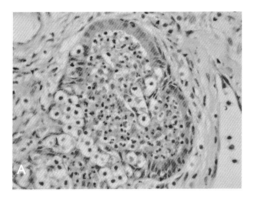

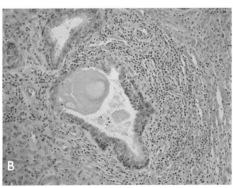

Prostatitis is also a histological condition, with inflammatory cells present within the prostatic ducts (A) and in the stroma in the periductal area (B)

A history lesson: 100 years of progress

Perhaps prostatitis is not always an infectious disease

Other therapies were introduced in the mid-1900s, including direct injection of antibiotics and other antiseptics directly into the urethra or prostate, introduction of novel anti-toxin therapies, application of heat and electrical therapy, and standardization of repetitive prostate massage. In 1968, Ed Meares and Thomas Stamey introduced their four-glass method of segmental localization of bacteria in the lower male urinary tract. Based on this and subsequent studies it was determined that uropathogenic bacteria could be identified in approximately 5% of patients presenting with chronic prostatitis. While this was helpful in identifying patients who may respond to antibiotic therapy, this advance did little for the majority of patients who presented with symptoms of abacterial prostatitis. In 1978 Drach and his colleagues classified prostatitis as acute bacterial prostatitis, chronic bacterial prostatitis, non-bacterial prostatitis and prostatodynia. This classification is now referred to as the 'traditional' classification system.

A 'best evidence-based' strategy

Research undertaken over the last 5 years has radically changed the management of prostatitis. Definitions and classifications of the disease based on international consensus, population-based epidemiological studies, application of molecular biological techniques, etiologic studies, evaluation of large cohorts of both prostatitis patients and asymptomatic control men, natural history studies and multi-center randomized placebo-controlled treatment trials are now allowing physicians to adopt a 'best evidence-based' strategy for diagnosing, categorizing and treating patients who present to them with prostatitis symptoms.

THE PROBLEM WITH PROSTATITIS
A HISTORY LESSON: 100 YEARS OF PROGRESS
Perhaps prostatitis is not always an infectious disease
A 'best evidence-based' strategy

Historic Time Line

350 BC	Prostate gland first described
1815	Inflammation of prostate described
1838	Pathology of prostatitis described
1893	Prostatitis as a clinical entity
1906	Microscopy of EPS
1913	Culture of EPS
1926	Role of bacteria confirmed
1927	Bacterial localisation studies
1928	Intraprostatic reflux described
1936	Prostate massage to obtain specimens
1938	Role of lower urinary tract obstruction
1957	Inflammation can be a non-bacterial process
1961	10-15 WBC/HPF – the Gold standard for EPS inflammation
1967	Poor correlation of symptoms, histology, WBC counts and EPS culture described
1968	Meares and Stamey 4-glass test
1978	Traditional classification system
1995	NIH classification system
1999	NIH chronic prostatitis symptom index

A historic time line illustrating advances in the understanding of prostatitis

13

Suggested reading

Drach GW, Fair WR, Meares EM, Stamey TA. Classification of benign diseases associated with prostatic pain: prostatitis or prostatodynia? J Urol 1978; 120: 266.

McNaughton-Collins M, Stafford RS, O'Leary MP, Barry MJ. How common is prostatitis? A national survey of physician visits. J Urol 1998; 159: 1224–1228.

Meares EM Jr, Stamey TA. Bacteriologic localization patterns in bacterial prostatitis and urethritis. Invest Urol 1968; 5: 492–518.

Moon TD. Questionnaire survey of urologists and primary care physicians' diagnostic and treatment practices for prostatitis. Urology 1997; 50: 543–547.

Nickel AC. The bacteriology of chronic prostatitis and seminal vesiculitis and elective localization of the bacteria as isolated. J Urol 1930; 24: 343–357.

Nickel JC. Prostatitis: an historic perspective. In: Nickel JC (ed) Textbook of Prostatatitis. Oxford: Isis Medical Media, 1999: 3–17.

Nickel JC, Nigro M, Valiquette L et al. Diagnosis and treatment of prostatitis in Canada. Urology 1998; 52: 797–802.

Nickel JC, Downey J, Hunter D, Clark J. Prevalance of prostatitis-like symptoms in a population based study employing the NIH-chronic prostatitis symptom index (NIH-CPSI). J Urol 2001; 165: 842.

Roberts RO, Lieber MM, Rhodes T, Girman CJ, Bostwick DG, Jacobsen SJ. Prevalence of a physician-assigned diagnosis of prostatitis: the Olmsted County Study of Urinary Symptoms and Health Status Among Men. Urology 1998; 51: 578–584.

Von Lackum WH. The infected prostate. Proc Staff Meetings Mayo Clinic 1928; 3: 14–16.

Wenninger K, Heiman JR, Rothman I, Berghuis JP, Berger RE. Sickness impact of chronic nonbacterial prostatitis and its correlates. J Urol 1996; 155: 965–968.

CHAPTER 2
ETIOLOGY OF PROSTATITIS: WHAT DO WE REALLY KNOW?

While many readers will skip this section and go directly to evaluation and treatment, it is important to understand what might be causing the patient's symptoms before one can rationalize the diagnostic and treatment plans outlined later in this manual. Current diagnostic and treatment strategies are based on what we know about the etiology of prostatitis. The confusion and frustration surrounding the management of this syndrome arise because of the gaps in our knowledge about the etiology; while future directions in research on the pathogenesis and etiology of the condition will ultimately lead to the key to better amelioration of symptoms and perhaps eventual cure.

INFECTIOUS

Historical record

Since the discovery of infectious diseases by Pasteur and others in the early twentieth century, microbial infection has been the most popular proposed etiologic mechanism for most kinds of inflammation, including prostatitis. While there was no doubt in any clinician's mind that generalized bacterial infection of the prostate – and for that matter the entire lower urinary tract – is responsible for signs and symptoms of acute bacterial prostatitis, the role of micro-organisms in the chronic syndrome is essentially unclear. Sophisticated localization techniques employed in the 1920s and 1930s identified and localized bacteria to the prostate glands of men suffering from prostatitis. Most of the organisms localized were not uropathogens as we know them today but rather gram-positive organisms such as *Streptococcus* and *Staphylococcus* species, which for many years in the latter part of the century were believed to be non-pathogenic. It was believed that these were either commensal organisms in the lower urinary tract or contaminants resulting from poor specimen collection or culture techniques. However, recent studies have confirmed that these gram-positive organisms can in fact be localized to the prostate gland, but their role in the pathogenesis of inflammation and symptoms is controversial. For instance, *Staphylococcus saprophyticus*, once thought to be a non-uropathogenic organism, is now believed to be responsible for a significant percentage of acute bacterial cystitis in sexually active young women. Could the same type of organisms be responsible for prostatic inflammation and symptoms? Uropathogenic bacteria such as gram-negative Enterobacteriaceae (*Escherichia coli, Klebsiella* spp., *Pseudomonas* spp., etc.) or presumed gram-positive uropathogens such as enterococci can also be localized to the prostate gland by employing careful standard lower urinary tract localization techniques. While there is no doubt that these uropathogenic organisms can be a nidus for lower

ETIOLOGY OF PROSTATITIS
INFECTIOUS
Historical record
Do bacteria cause the symptoms?
Other micro-organisms

urinary tract infections (i.e. recurrent cystitis), it is difficult to prove that their existence in the prostate is related to the patient's symptoms.

Do bacteria cause the symptoms?

A recent report on a large cohort of chronic prostatitis/chronic pelvic pain syndrome patients by the NIH Chronic Prostatitis Collaborative Research Network confirmed that the presence or absence of uropathogenic bacteria, or for that matter any bacteria, did not correlate with symptoms. In fact, prostatic inflammation, measured by the degree of leukocytosis in prostate specific specimens, also did not correlate with symptoms. Furthermore, studies performed in the late 1950s and early 1960s on asymptomatic control patients suggested that normal asymptomatic men without clinical prostatitis may have both uropathogenic and presumed non-uropathogenic bacteria localized to the prostate gland. A recent large study of over 120 control patients by the NIH Chronic Prostatitis Collaborative Research Network confirms this finding. Numerous studies, which cultured prostatic tissue removed during transurethral resection of the prostate in men with benign prostatic hyperplasia (BPH), also confirm the presence of bacteria within the prostate gland of men without clinical prostatitis. Bacteria are present in the prostate gland of men with chronic prostatitis, and while they may be important in the acute initiation of symptoms, their role in the chronic symptomatology remains unknown.

Other micro-organisms

Bacteria are not the only organisms found in the lower urinary tract. Chlamydia (*Chlamydia trachomatis*) and mycoplasma (*Ureaplasma urealyticum*) are responsible for non-specific urethritis in men. It would seem obvious that organisms that cause urethral inflammation can potentially reflux into the prostate gland, and if the conditions are right, create a scenario for inflammation in and around the prostatic ducts and acini. Studies have shown that chronic prostatitis patients, particularly those with definite inflammation of the prostate gland, have a higher prevalence of these organisms in urethral specimens and prostate specific specimens. Biopsy studies of the prostate and utilization of sophisticated molecular biological techniques such as polymerase chain reaction (PCR) have also identified these organisms, as well as a number of unusual species of micro-organisms within the prostate. However, these findings are not universal and other equally well designed and carried out studies have either not found the same prevalence of these organisms within prostate specific specimens or have found similar prevalence of these organisms in asymptomatic control men. Other micro-organisms such as fungi and viruses have also been implicated in the initiation and propagation of prostatic inflammation. However, the proof that these organisms may be implicated in chronic prostatitis in men who are not immunocompromised (i.e. with HIV infection or immunosuppression medication) is very slim.

Previous history of infection

Many patients presenting with a long history of chronic prostatitis symptoms will recollect an initial episode that sounds infectious in nature, either urethritis or cystitis. Sometimes this is documented but many times it is not. Many of these patients also report an initial resolution or at least improvement in their symptoms with antibiotics, usually given for only short periods of time for such an acute event. It has been hypothesized that if the bacteria are not eradicated at initial presentation, the bacteria

ETIOLOGY OF PROSTATITIS
INFECTIOUS
Other micro-organisms
Previous history of infection

develop a protective mode of survival within the prostate gland itself. This bacterial self-preservation mechanism, called bacterial biofilm formation, involves microcolonies or aggregates of bacteria adherent to the ductal and acinar walls, secreting an exopolysaccharide slime in which they exist in a low activity state (almost hibernating). This decreased metabolic state and protective 'glycocalyx' coating protects the biofilm bacteria from host defenses and antibiotics. Unknown triggers allow the bacteria to come out of this state, replicate and through immune mechanisms promote recurrent and chronic inflammation. Such bacterial biofilms have been found in electron microscopy studies of biopsy specimens. This theory would also explain why bacteria can be grown in biopsy specimens and detected by molecular biological techniques when they cannot be grown in the prostatic fluid or semen. It might also explain the recent finding that more bacteria can be detected by culturing specimens for 5 days instead of the standard 2 days.

Infectious agents possibly implicated in the pathogenesis of prostatitis.

Uropathogenic bacteria	*Escherichia coli, Klebsiella* spp., *Pseudomonas* spp., other Enterobacteriaceae
Probable prostate pathogens	Enterococci
Possible prostate pathogens	*Chlamydia* spp., *Mycoplasma* spp., anaerobic bacteria, *Corynebacterium* spp., 'biofilm bacteria'
Potential prostate pathogens	Fungi (*Candida* spp.) Viruses Other cryptic non-culturable micro-organisms

Previous history of infection

The largely popular micro-organism-based theory of prostatitis pathogenesis is the key to the common employment of antimicrobial therapy in chronic prostatitis patients, even those with negative cultures.

Bacteria threatened by environmental forces (in the case of prostatitis, antibiotics or host defenses) tend to aggregate on surfaces (the prostatic duct wall), envelope themselves with a slime layer (an exopolysaccharide or 'glycocalyx' produced by the bacteria) and reduce their metabolic activity (almost hibernate). This mode of existence protects them from antibiotics and host defenses while allowing the bacteria to promote a low grade immunologic reaction. Under certain circumstances the bacteria become active again, reproduce and cause recurrent urinary tract infections.

The electron micrograph show an aggregate of bacteria in prostatic duct

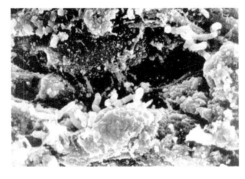

Bacteria adhere to the interstices and surfaces of prostate calculi, making them very difficult to eradicate with antibiotic therapy

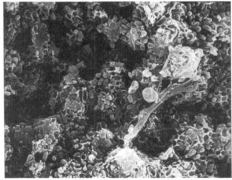

ANATOMIC

It is believed that two major anatomic abnormalities may play a role in the initiation and propagation of prostatitis: obstruction and reflux. Obstruction of the lower urinary tract caused by either bladder neck hyperplasia, benign prostatic hyperplasia, external sphincter dyssynergia, urethral stricture, meatal stenosis or even phimosis can cause high pressure dysfunctional voiding. The high pressure turbulence caused by such obstruction changes the flow characteristics of urine through the urethra, creating currents and back eddies that can literally drag bacteria from the distal urethra into the area of the prostatic urethra. If the patient's personal prostatic anatomy is associated with a less acute insertion of the prostatic duct into the prostatic urethra, a potential scenario exists for intra-prostatic reflux. Urine with potentially harmful and toxic constituents (potassium, immunogenic proteins, etc.) and/or micro-organisms passing through or dragged into the prostatic urethra, can reflux into the prostatic ducts and even the acini. Prostatic ductal architecture is such that the peri-urethral area and the peripheral gland would be involved first, which appears to be the case in the pathogenesis of prostatic inflammation. This theory for the initiation of prostatic inflammation and subsequent symptoms would explain the benefits of a number of medical (e.g. alpha-blockers, finasteride) and surgical (e.g. incision of the bladder neck) therapies.

21

Anatomic

Voiding
cystourethrograms
in patients with
obstructive voiding
due to vesical-
sphincter
dyssnynergia (A)
and bladder neck
obstruction (B)
showing
intraprostatic reflux

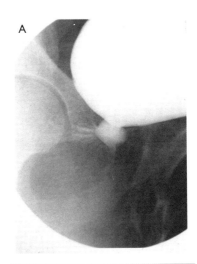

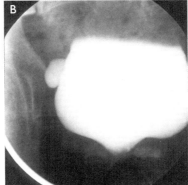

TRAUMATIC

For over a century now, and probably since antiquity, patients and physicians have recognized that repetitive perineal trauma results in chronic perineal and pelvic pain. This was first described in medical literature with patients experiencing chronic perineal pain associated with horseback riding or riding on hard, wooden seats in poorly suspended buggies. This has been described more recently in long-distance bicycle riders, and clinicians are generally aware of this syndrome occurring in many truck, tractor and heavy equipment drivers. Most probably, this repetitive trauma affects the local perineal muscle and nervous system,

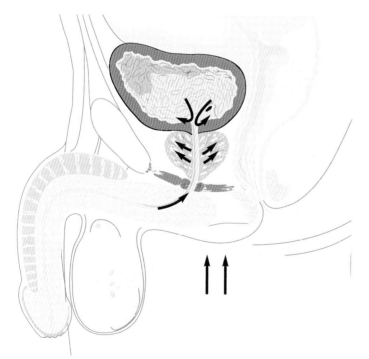

The prostatitis syndrome likely begins with a specific initiator which causes acute (and repetitive) perineal/pelvic injury or acute followed by sub-acute and chronic inflammation

perhaps even the vascular system (i.e. local ischemia). The author has even hypothesized that if the perineum is thought of as a limb, repetitive perineal trauma may result in a local reflex sympathetic dystrophy syndrome. This would explain the muscular, neurogenic and perhaps even vascular symptoms and signs associated with this variant of chronic prostatitis/chronic pelvic pain syndrome. It also suggests various avenues of treatment, primarily avoidance of potentially traumatic experiences.

IMMUNOLOGIC

Bacteria, toxic substances in the urine or any other proposed etiological agent arriving in the prostate gland could not cause inflammation without initiating an immune reaction. While the immune system is unlikely to be the initiator of the events leading to prostatic inflammation and subsequent symptoms, it certainly is intimately involved in the pathogenesis and propagation of the inflammation. The immunologic cascade, propagated by cytokine activation and inflammatory cell infiltration, is stimulated either by specific receptors associated with the bacterial surface or by non-specific stimulation by chemical or other irritant factors. Evidence has accumulated that this scenario may turn into an autoimmune process, such that continued chronic inflammation is propagated by autoimmune mechanisms, even when the initiating agent has been eradicated, resolved or has disappeared.

This hypothesis on the role of the immune system for the pathogenesis and propagation of chronic prostatic inflammation suggests many sites along the immunologic cascade for therapeutic intervention. This, of course, is the rationale for the use of anti-inflammatory and immunosuppressive agents.

NEUROMUSCULAR

The symptoms experienced by patients suffering from chronic prostatitis eventually develop into a typical neuropathic pain pattern, with associated local muscular dysfunction. It is unlikely that the dysregulation of the pelvic neurologic system is a primary mechanism but rather a result of preceding causes. This is discussed in the next section.

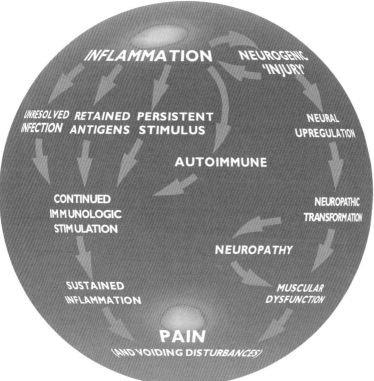

Inflammation and neurogenic injury can be propagated by autoimmune processes or upregulation of the local neural loop. Chronic neuropathy can promote a neurogenically mediated inflammation while chronic inflammation can promote further neurologic injury

25

INTERSTITIAL CYSTITIS

Interstitial cystitis is a chronic pelvic pain syndrome characterized by urinary frequency, urgency, and bladder pain (usually relieved by voiding). This cystitis-like syndrome, which occurs most commonly in women, is not associated with demonstrable infection with typical uropathogenic bacteria. It has been hypothesized that men with chronic pelvic pain may have the same etiologic mechanisms and pathogenic processes but further complicated by having a prostate gland. In fact, a review of the proposed etiologies for interstitial cystitis reveals many of the same infectious, traumatic, anatomic (or physiologic), immunologic, and neurogenic mechanisms proposed for chronic prostatitis. Similarly the treatments suggested for interstitial cystitis and chronic prostatitis are almost identical. It is very likely that the chronic pelvic pain and associated voiding symptoms of interstitial cystitis and chronic prostatitis exist along the same etiological and pathogenic spectrum.

A MULTIFACTORIAL INTER-RELATED CASCADE – THE FINAL PATHWAY

It became quite evident to the author and many other researchers that chronic prostatitis/chronic pelvic pain syndrome is not secondary to a single, defined etiologic agent, but rather a syndrome consisting of a continuous spectrum, initiated and propagated by multiple, likely inter-related factors. The author's opinion is that patients with chronic prostatitis/chronic pelvic pain syndrome may have any number of factors initiating an acute event. These 'initiators' could be infection, high pressure dysfunctional voiding, trauma, or some unknown toxin. This initiating event results in either injury and/or inflammation. The injury could be to the local nerves and muscles or even the prostatic glandular or stromal tissue. Inflammation likely is initially restricted to the prostate and peri-prostatic area. The initial neuropathy or immunologic reaction can progress because of persistent initiating factors (persistence of bacteria, dysfunctional voiding or perineal trauma). However, the neuropathic and immunologic pathology could persist, even with eradication or amelioration of the initiating factor, through a self-perpetuating stimulatory loop. Inflammation can continue because of initiation of a new autoimmune mechanism. Inflammation in the prostatic and peri-prostatic area can promote a neurogenic reaction resulting in chronic neuropathy. It is also recognized that peripheral neuropathy can initiate and promote a progressive and durable inflammatory reaction. Upregulation of the local pelvic neural loop perpetuates the neuropathic state. The result for the patient is pain in the perineum, pelvis and genitalia, abnormal voiding parameters and because of the proximity of the erectile mechanisms in the area, various degrees of sexual dysfunction. Unfortunately, this is the state at which most of the patients with chronic prostatitis/chronic pelvic pain syndrome present, at least to the urologic specialist. Therapies aimed at the initiating factors are important to eradicate potentiating agents; however, in the long term, they may prove ineffective, because the syndrome has progressed along the spectrum of disease where the initiating event may now be irrelevant. This is the rationale for the introduction of neurologic medications, neuromodulatory interventions and physical therapies.

KEY POINT

■ Prostatitis represents a spectrum that begins with an inter-related multifactorial cascade of events that culminates in a final pathway producing pain, voiding and sexual disturbances. Various initiators cause local inflammation or neurogenic injury which propagates by autoimmune processes or up-regulation of local neural loops, creating an inter-related scenario of chronic inflammation and chronic neuropathy

27

Suggested reading

Berger RE, Krieger JN, Rothman I, Muller CH, Hillier SL. Bacteria in the prostate tissue of men with idiopathic prostatic inflammation. J Urol 1997; 157: 863–865.

Blacklock NJ. The anatomy of the prostate: relationship with prostatic infection. Infection 1991; 19: S111–S114.

Doble A. The diagnosis, aetiology and pathogenesis of chronic non-bacterial prostatitis. In: Nickel JC (ed) Textbook of Prostatitis. Oxford: Isis Medical Media, 1999: 123–127.

Domingue GJ. Cryptic bacterial infection in chronic prostatitis: diagnostic and therapeutic implications. Curr Opin Urol 1998; 8: 45–49.

Nickel JC. Prostatitis: an infectious disease? Infections in Urology 2000; 13: 31–38.

Nickel JC, MacLean RJL. Bacterial biofilms in urology. Infections in Urology 1998; 11: 168–175.

Sant GR, Nickel JC. Interstitial cystitis in chronic prostatitis: the same syndrome? Nickel JC (ed) Textbook of Prostatitis. Oxford: Isis Medical Media, 1999: 169–176.

Shoskes DA, Moody JA. Prostatodynia. In: Nickel JC (ed) Textbook of Prostatitis. Oxford: Isis Medical Media, 1999: 149–156.

Zermann DH, Schmidt RA. Neurophysiology of the pelvic floor: its role in prostate and pelvic pain. In: Nickel JC (ed) Textbook of Prostatitis. Oxford: Isis Medical Media, 1999: 95–105.

CHAPTER 3
EVALUATION OF THE PROSTATITIS PATIENT: THE FIRST STEP IN MANAGEMENT

The first step in understanding how to evaluate the patient presenting with chronic prostatitis is to realize that this condition is not a disease, but rather a syndrome. The patient presents with a constellation of symptoms along a wide and very variable spectrum of possible presentations. Numerous studies, however, have confirmed that the primary symptom is that of pain. The pain can be localized anywhere in the genitourinary tract or pelvis but the primary six locations or types of pain include the perineum, suprapubic area, groin/testicles, penis and pain or discomfort associated with ejaculation or voiding. A secondary but important associated consideration is that of irritative and obstructive voiding symptoms; frequency, urgency, nocturia, hesitancy, poor stream and a feeling of inadequate bladder emptying. Symptoms of sexual dysfunction can also be important in some patients but in most series, other than the major symptom of ejaculatory pain and discomfort, sexual disturbances do not play a major role. This constellation of symptoms, which is highly variable in number, frequency and severity, severely impacts on a patient's quality of life. This impact can range from a mild nuisance to moderately or severely limiting the life activities and experiences of the patient. The other two main factors or parameters that are important in the diagnosis are evaluation of bacteria and inflammation in the lower urinary tract. These are accomplished by employing some form of lower urinary tract specimen sampling for microscopy (looking for white blood cells and other clues of inflammation) and culture (determining the local bacterial flora of the lower urinary tract). All other investigations are employed to exclude other causes for the patient's presenting symptoms.

CLASSIFICATION SYSTEM FOR CLINICAL PRACTICE

It is generally accepted that there is a definite and defined bacterial etiology in acute bacterial prostatitis and for the recurrent urinary tract infections in chronic bacterial prostatitis. However, in the majority of patients, the symptoms do not present acutely with bacterial cystitis and lower urinary tract infection. Furthermore most patients do not have recurrent urinary tract infections nor does the physician find uropathogenic bacteria on culturing prostate specific specimens. In the past these patients (from whose specimens no uropathogenic bacteria are cultured) were either categorized as chronic non-bacterial or abacterial prostatitis if inflammation was noted on the expressed prostatic secretion or alternatively as prostatodynia, if no inflammation was noted on expressed prostatic secretion. It was recognized late in the 1990s by a consensus group convened by the National Institutes of Health in Washington that even if these symptoms originated in the prostate, by the time most patients presented, the prostate may not be the primary organ involved. Many believe that the syndrome is caused by a neuromuscular problem in the perineum and pelvic floor or alternatively a bladder or entire lower urinary tract dysfunction. For this reason it was felt that it was inappropriate to label these patients as having a prostate problem by diagnosing prostatitis or prostatodynia. It is believed by many that this has led to the confusion we have seen in the field for the last several decades and perhaps inappropriate prostate-directed therapies. It was decided at this meeting to develop a new classification system for prostatitis that would be appropriate for use in research and clinical studies but also be practical for use in clinical practice.

This new National Institutes of Health prostatitis classification included four main categories. Category I or acute bacterial prostatitis is associated with an acute, generalized infection of the prostate gland. Category II or chronic bacterial prostatitis is diagnosed by demonstrating uropathogenic bacteria in the culture of prostate specific specimens. Category II prostatitis is characterized by recurrent urinary tract infections with the same organism. Chronic non-bacterial prostatitis and prostatodynia would now be called Category III chronic pelvic pain syndrome (or CPPS). Patients diagnosed with CPPS would present with pain and/or discomfort in the pelvic region for longer than 3 months. Patients would be included in this category if no uropathogenic bacteria were localized to prostate specific specimens (expressed prostatic secretion, post-prostatic massage urine or semen) on culture. This category is further subdivided into an inflammatory group (Category IIIA CPPS) and non-inflammatory group (Category IIIB CPPS), based on the degree of leukocytosis (number of white blood cells) in the prostate specific specimens. Studies have indicated that >95% of patients presenting with chronic prostatitis would be included in this category. The NIH classification also included a unique and very interesting new category, Category IV or asymptomatic inflammatory prostatitis (AIP). Patients diagnosed with Category IV AIP are asymptomatic and the inflammation noted on prostate specific specimens or histologic preparations is usually an incidental finding in patients being assessed for elevated PSA, benign prostatic hyperplasia or infertility. Some feel that this category of prostatitis may hold the key, not only to prostatic inflammation but also to the other major prostate diseases, benign prostatic hyperplasia and prostate cancer.

Traditional Classification System	National Institutes of Health Classification System	Description	Presentation
Acute bacterial prostatitis	Category I	Acute infection of the prostate gland	Acute febrile illness associated with perineal and suprapubic pain, dysuria, and obstructive voiding symptoms
Chronic bacterial prostatitis	Category II	Chronic infection of the prostate	Recurrent urinary tract infections (usually with same organism) associated frequently with voiding disturbances
Non-bacterial prostatitis/ prostatodynia	Category III Chronic pelvic pain syndrome (CPPS)	Chronic genito-urinary pain in the absence of uropathogenic bacteria localized to the prostate gland employing standard methodology	Chronic perineal, suprapubic, groin, testicular, penile, ejaculatory pain associated with variable dysuria and obstructive and irritative voiding symptoms
	Category IIIA Inflammatory CPPS	Significant number of white blood cells in expressed prostatic secretions, post-prostatic massage urine sediment (VB3) or semen	
	Category IIIB Non-inflammatory CPPS	Insignificant number of white blood cells in expressed prostatic secretions, post-prostatic massage urine sediment (VB3) or semen	
	Category IV Asymptomatic inflammatory prostatitis (AIP)	White blood cells (and/ or bacteria) in expressed prostatic secretions, post-prostatic massage urine sediment (VB3), semen or histological specimens of prostate gland	Asymptomatic

EVALUATION OF THE PROSTATITIS PATIENT
CLASSIFICATION SYSTEM FOR CLINICAL PRACTICE
CLINICAL DIAGNOSIS
Acute bacterial prostatitis (Category I)
Chronic bacterial prostatitis (Category II)

CLINICAL DIAGNOSIS

Acute bacterial prostatitis (Category I)

Patients with acute bacterial prostatitis present with acute local and systemic symptoms, which usually include severe perineal and suprapubic pain, irritative and obstructive voiding symptoms associated with dysuria and in most cases fever and generalized aches and pains. The prostate is usually boggy (soft) and exquisitely tender on examination, as is the perineum and suprapubic area on palpation. These symptoms and signs reflect the pathogenesis of this particular category of prostatitis, that of a bacterial infection of the prostate and in most cases the entire lower urinary tract. Clinical assessment would then include a history of the relevant symptoms and a physical examination – which would of course include examination of the abdomen, external genitalia, perineum and a digital rectal examination. Before treatment is instituted, mid-stream culture of urine is mandatory. If the patient is very ill it is usually a good idea to obtain blood cultures as well.

Chronic bacterial prostatitis (Category II)

Patients with chronic bacterial prostatitis may not be symptomatic between acute flare-ups. This diagnosis is characterized by recurrent urinary tract infections, usually with the same organism. Following successful antibiotic therapy, many, but not all, of these patients become asymptomatic. Bacteria can be localized to prostate specific specimens (expressed prostatic secretion, post-prostatic massage urine and/or semen) using the diagnostic methods outlined later in this chapter. For the most part, physical examination including digital rectal examination may be entirely non-contributory to the diagnosis.

Chronic non-bacterial prostatitis/prostatodynia (Category III Chronic pelvic pain syndrome)

Since chronic prostatitis/chronic pelvic pain syndrome (CP/CPPS) is a syndrome, it is best diagnosed and characterized by the constellation of symptoms with which it is associated. Therefore the diagnosis of CP/CPPS is a clinical diagnosis in patients without clinical or culture documented infection. There are no objective signs or laboratory tests that would definitively differentiate a CP/CPPS patient from a normal male without symptomatic prostatitis. Clinically, these patients have a long history (certainly 3 months or longer) of genitourinary and pelvic pain, irritative and obstructive voiding symptoms, perhaps some symptoms of sexual dysfunction and often other associated generalized symptoms such as fatigue or 'aches and pains'. Except for eliciting pain in various trigger points in the pelvis, perineum or external genitalia, the physical examination does not usually contribute much information. The prostate usually feels normal but can feel soft or 'boggy'. In most cases palpation of the prostate does elicit tenderness but the same tenderness can be noted on vigorous prostatic massage in normal asymptomatic men. The primary importance of the physical examination is to rule out other causes of pain and discomfort and to produce and collect prostate specific specimens (such as expressed prostatic secretion).

A SYMPTOM ASSESSMENT TOOL

It has always been very difficult to assess the symptomatology
in patients presenting with chronic prostatitis. The difficulty is not only
in comparing severity of symptoms between patients but also in following
frequency, severity and impact of symptoms over time. This is illustrated
most importantly in most of the prostatitis treatment studies published
over the last several decades. With no standardized assessment of
symptoms, the success of therapy became extremely subjective and it was
impossible to compare the results of one treatment trial with another.
Recognizing the need for a practical, validated and reliable symptom
assessment tool in chronic prostatitis, the National Institutes of Health
Chronic Prostatitis Collaborative Research Network undertook a large-
scale study to determine whether such a tool could be developed. The
NIH/Chronic Prostatitis Symptom Index (NIH-CPSI) was developed out
of this exhaustive study. It was discovered that the prostatitis experience
could be adequately explored by examining the pain and discomfort of
symptoms (location, frequency and severity), the irritative and obstructive
voiding symptoms and the impact of these symptoms on the patient's
quality of life. Nine separate items that could be answered by most
patients in about 5 minutes addressed all these important issues. The six
major locations or type of pain or discomfort, the frequency of pain or
discomfort and severity of pain or discomfort were rated on a scale of
0–21. The irritative and obstructive voiding symptoms were rated on a
score of 0–10 while the impact on quality of life was rated on a score of
0–12. Each of these domains could be assessed independently or the three
could be added together for a total NIH-CPSI score of 0–43.

The NIH-CPSI has proved to be invaluable in prostatitis research. It has
allowed us to proceed with large epidemiological studies, longitudinal
natural history studies of patients with chronic prostatitis, comparisons of
chronic prostatitis patients and patients with no prostatitis and has

A symptom assessment tool

allowed us to develop clinical treatment trials with a valid outcome parameter. But even more important, the NIH-CPSI has proved itself as a valuable tool for the practicing urologist. The urologist should have the patient fill out the NIH-CPSI at the first visit, along with a simple form for demographics and medical history. The physician can then quickly assess the completed index and will be able to focus the interview on the points that the patient feels are most important. The patient is gratified that the physician understands his concerns and problems and the physician finds the clinical encounter to be much less frustrating. Along with the lower urinary tract evaluation (later in this chapter) the physician can use the NIH-CPSI to obtain a baseline yardstick by which the patient's progress can be measured over time. As will be illustrated in the treatment section, it is rare to cure patients with chronic prostatitis syndrome (perhaps Mother Nature cures them while we are entertaining them) and the NIH-CPSI can be used to confirm improvement of symptoms over time; degrees of amelioration of symptoms that the patients may not be able to appreciate because they occur so slowly. The physician can quickly judge on subsequent visits whether the recommended treatment was successful or should be abandoned for another approach. This leads to considerably less confusion and frustration for both patient and physician in the management of the chronic prostatitis syndromes.

KEY POINT

■ The National Institutes of Health Chronic Prostatitis Symptom Index (NIH-CPSI) captures the 3 most important domains of the prostatitis experience: pain, voiding and quality of life. This index is useful in research studies and clinical practice.

NIH-Chronic Prostatitis Symptom Index (NIH-CPSI)

Pain or Discomfort

1. In the last week, have you experienced any pain or discomfort in the following areas?

	Yes	No
a. Area between rectum and testicles (perineum)	❏ 1	❏ 0
b. Testicles	❏ 1	❏ 0
c. Tip of the penis (not related to urination)	❏ 1	❏ 0
d. Below your waist, in your pubic or bladder area	❏ 1	❏ 0

2. In the last week, have you experienced:

	Yes	No
a. Pain or burning during urination?	❏ 1	❏ 0
b. Pain or discomfort during or after sexual climax (ejaculation)?	❏ 1	❏ 0

3. How often have you had pain or discomfort in any of these areas over the last week?

❏ 0 Never
❏ 1 Rarely
❏ 2 Sometimes
❏ 3 Often
❏ 4 Usually
❏ 5 Always

4. Which number best describes your AVERAGE pain or discomfort on the days that you had it, over the last week?

❏	❏	❏	❏	❏	❏	❏	❏	❏	❏	❏
0	1	2	3	4	5	6	7	8	9	10

NO PAIN   PAIN AS BAD AS YOU CAN IMAGINE

Urination

5. How often have you had a sensation of not emptying your bladder completely after you finished urinating, over the last week?

❏ 0 Not at all
❏ 1 Less than 1 time in 5
❏ 2 Less than half the time
❏ 3 About half the time
❏ 4 More than half the time
❏ 5 Almost always

6. How often have you had to urinate again less than two hours after you finished urinating, over the last week?

❏ 0 Not at all
❏ 1 Less than 1 time in 5
❏ 2 Less than half the time
❏ 3 About half the time
❏ 4 More than half the time
❏ 5 Almost always

Impact of Symptoms

7. How much have your symptoms kept you from doing the kinds of things you would usually do, over the last week?

❏ 0 None
❏ 1 Only a little
❏ 2 Some
❏ 3 A lot

8. How much did you think about your symptoms, over the last week?

❏ 0 None
❏ 1 Only a little
❏ 2 Some
❏ 3 A lot

Quality of Life

9. If you were to spend the rest of your life with your symptoms just the way they have been during the last week, how would you feel about that?

❏ 0 Delighted
❏ 1 Pleased
❏ 2 Mostly satisfied
❏ 3 Mixed (about equally satisfied and dissatisfied)
❏ 4 Mostly dissatisfied
❏ 5 Unhappy
❏ 6 Terrible

Scoring the NIH-Chronic Prostatitis Symptom Index Domains

Pain: Total of items 1a, 1b, 1c, 1d, 2a, 2b, 3, and 4 = ___

Urinary Symptoms: Total of items 5 and 6 = ___

Quality of Life Impact: Total of items 7, 8, and 9 = ___

The National Institutes of Health Chronic Prostatitis Symptom Index (courtesy of Litwin MS, McNaughton-Collins M, Fowler FJ et al. The NIH Chronic Prostatitis Symptom Index (NIH-CPSI): development and validation of a new outcome measure. J Urol 1999; 162: 369–337; with permission).

A SIMPLE LOWER URINARY TRACT LOCALIZATION TECHNIQUE

The Meares-Stamey 4-glass lower urinary tract localization test was described in 1968. The original description was based on very few patients and was never validated, yet it became the 'gold standard' for evaluation of prostatitis patients. A comprehensive description of this technique can be found in every major urology and infectious disease textbook published in the 1970s to the 1990s. Yet surveys of most physicians, including urologists, have shown unequivocally that it is not widely used in clinical practice.

The 4-glass test makes clinical sense. Bacteria or leukocytosis in the initial first voided specimen (VB1) indicates urethritis. Uropathogenic bacteria in the mid-stream urine specimen (VB2) would indicate that the patient has either primary or associated cystitis. Uropathogenic bacteria in the expressed prostatic secretion or post-prostatic massage urine specimen (VB3) would lead to a diagnosis of bacterial prostatitis, if the same bacteria were not present (or cultured in a 100-fold less concentration) in the VB1 and VB2. In patients in whom no uropathogenic bacteria are cultured, the presence of white blood cells in the expressed prostatic secretion (EPS) or post-prostatic massage urine sediment (VB3) would mean that the patient had prostatic inflammation – non-bacterial or abacterial prostatitis. No demonstrable inflammation on microscopy in otherwise sterile prostate specific specimens would indicate that the patient had a sterile, non-inflamed prostate and would therefore be diagnosed with prostatodynia. However, physicians did not perform this test unless the patients were in clinical research trials. The reasons are many: the test is cumbersome, expensive, difficult, and most importantly, rarely appeared to change any therapeutic decision-making.

But a physician cannot just prescribe treatment without any type of lower tract evaluation. The pre- and post-massage test was introduced so that physicians could perform an adequate evaluation of the culture and inflammatory status of the lower urinary tract without resorting to a cumbersome, expensive test. A mid-stream urine specimen is taken and sent to the laboratory for culture and microscopy of the sediment. Vigorous prostatic massage is performed and the initial stream of urine after prostatic massage (post-prostatic massage urine) is also sent as a separate specimen for culture and microscopic examination of the sediment. Uropathogenic bacteria localized to the post-prostatic specimen indicate bacterial presence within the prostate and a subsequent diagnosis of Category II prostatitis. In patients with no uropathogenic growth in

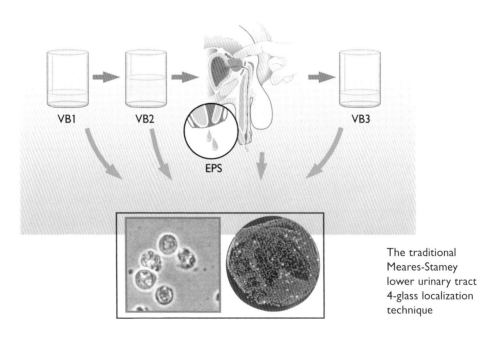

The traditional Meares-Stamey lower urinary tract 4-glass localization technique

A simple lower urinary tract localization technique

the specimens, the presence of a significant number of white blood cells (no one has confirmed the appropriate cut-off point but it is probably between 5 and 10 WBC/HPF) in the post-prostatic massage urine specimen would indicate prostatic inflammation and a subsequent diagnosis of Category IIIA CPPS. The absence of bacteria or white blood cells would lead to a diagnosis of Category IIIB CPPS. Studies have shown that the pre- and post-massage test (2-glass PPMT) is not quite as accurate as the more rigorous Meares-Stamey 4-glass test. However, it is easier to perform and more cost-effective but still allows the physician to categorize the majority of patients presenting with chronic prostatitis appropriately.

The pre and post-prostatic massage 2-glass test

Pre-M

Post-M

The technique of prostatic massage

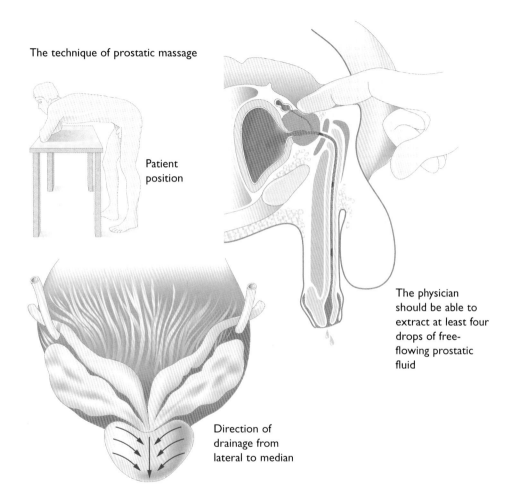

Patient position

The physician should be able to extract at least four drops of free-flowing prostatic fluid

Direction of drainage from lateral to median

KEY POINT

■ It is important to determine if uropathogenic bacteria can be localized to prostate specific specimens.

A simple lower urinary tract localization technique

CATEGORY II

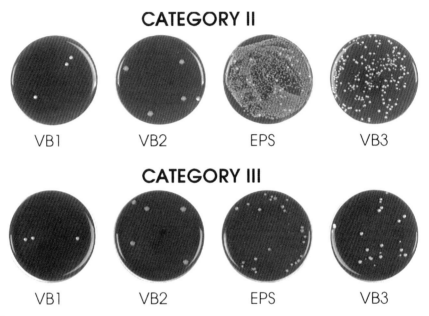

| VB1 | VB2 | EPS | VB3 |

CATEGORY III

| VB1 | VB2 | EPS | VB3 |

Typical culture plates seen in localization studies of patients with Category II and Category III CPPS

KEY POINT

■ It is important to document the degree of prostatic inflammation by employing some form of lower urinary tract localization study

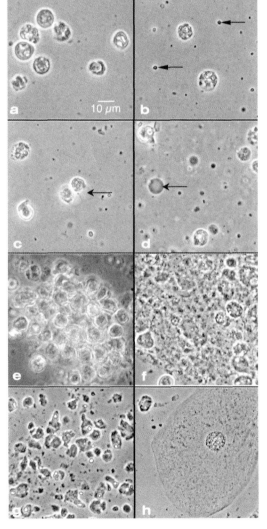

Photomicrographs of cells and particles often observed in wet mount preparations of expressed prostatic secretions.

a) Eight leukocytes, predominantly polymorphonuclear neutrophils. Slightly smaller irregular masses are isolated nuclei.

b) Lipid droplets of various sizes and densities (arrows) should not be counted as cells.

c) Occasionally cells (arrow) are in the process of losing the nucleus, probably as a result of pressure between the glass slide and coverslip.

d) Large lipid droplet or cytoplast (arrow) that is cytoplasm and cell membrane remaining after nucleus loss, are not counted as cells.

e) Clumped masses of cells in which accurate cell count is impossible.

f) Many cells trapped in amorphous matrix containing cells.

g) High concentration of degenerating leukocytes and small epithelial cells in a case of bacterial prostatitis.

h) Squamous epithelial cells which may have been contaminants from skin.

(From Muller CH, Berger RE, Mohr LE, Krieger JN. Comparison of microscopic methods for detecting inflammation in expressed prostatic secretions. J Urol 2001; 166: 2518–2524; reproduced with permission.)

A simple lower urinary tract localization technique

Bright field microscopy (×100 magnification, oil immersion objective) of cells typically found in expressed prostatic secretion smears. These cells have been stained.

a) Polymorphonuclear neutrophils are the most common cell type. Note typical bridges between nuclear lobes. Scale bar represents 10 μ.
b) Polymorphonuclear neutrophil, possibly at less mature stage as band neutrophil.
c) Monocyte or macrophage precursor.
d) Macrophage.
e) Macrophage with large phagocytic vacule causing signet ring appearance.
f) Eosinophil or eosinophilic band neutrophil with bilobate nucleus and red granules.
g) Squamous epithelial cell with numerous attached bacteria which are not rare on these cells and may not have clinical significance, since cells are likely skin contaminants.
h) Prostatic epithelial cells of various shapes are found due partially to natural variation and possibly to mechanics of producing fluid smear on slide.

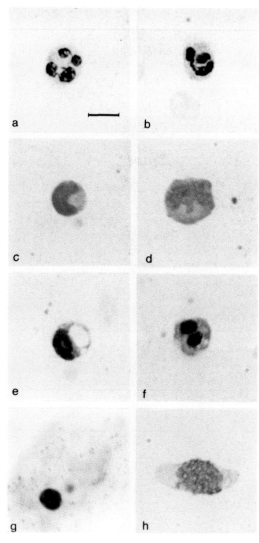

(From Muller CH, Berger RE, Mohr LE, Krieger JN. Comparison of microscopic methods for detecting inflammation in expressed prostatic secretions. J Urol 2001; 166: 2518-2524; reproduced with permission.)

Interpretation of the four-glass test (Meares-Stamey) and two-glass pre- and post-massage test (PPMT)

TEST		MEARES-STAMEY				PPMT	
SPECIMEN		VB1	VB2	EPS	VB3	Pre-M	Post-M
CAT II	WBC	–	+/–*	+	+	+/–*	+
	CULTURE	–	+/–*	+	+	+/–*	+
CAT IIIA	WBC	–	–	+	+	–	+
	CULTURE	–	–	–	–	–	–
CAT IIIB	WBC	–	–	–	–	–	–
	CULTURE	–	–	–	–	–	–

CAT   National Institute of Health Classification Category,

WBC   white blood cells,

VB1   first voided urine specimen,

VB2   second voided urine specimen or midstream specimen,

EPS   expressed prostatic secretion,

VB3   third voided urine specimen,

Pre-M   urine specimen before prostate massage,

Post-M   urine specimen after prostate massage,

*   Cystitis can co-exist with chronic bacterial prostatitis. If confirmation is required, repeat after 3 days of nitrofurantoin therapy.

OTHER TESTS

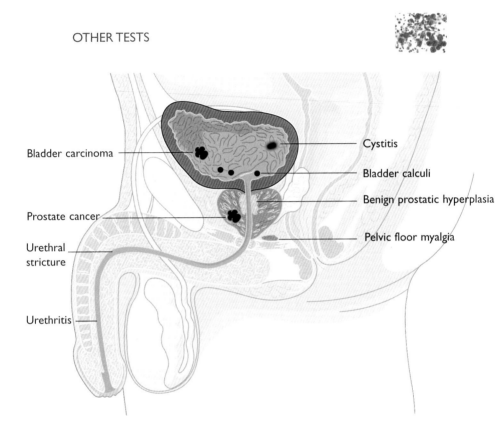

Bladder carcinoma

Prostate cancer

Urethral stricture

Urethritis

Cystitis

Bladder calculi

Benign prostatic hyperplasia

Pelvic floor myalgia

Other tests may be required to rule out causes for the patient's symptoms (differential diagnoses)

Semen analysis

The NIH classification system also employs the ejaculate specimen as a possible parameter to assess lower urinary tract infection and inflammation. Certainly the semen does contain some prostatic and seminal vesicular fluid, but studies comparing semen analysis and culture to expressed prostatic secretion (EPS) microscopy and culture have not shown a strong correlation. Similarly the leukocyte and bacterial status of the semen in normal men has not yet been fully elucidated. The microscopic examination of semen requires staining to identify white blood cells (which can look like immature sperm on unstained wet mount preparations). However, culture of semen does identify potentially uropathogenic bacteria in the lower urinary tract, as long as it is combined with initial stream urine culture (VB1) to rule out urethral colonization (which would show up in semen culture as well). Microscopy of the semen would also increase the number of patients who would be ultimately classified as Category IIIA, although the clinical significance of this is really unknown.

Urethral swab

Any patient who complains of urethral discharge, dysuria as the primary symptom or urethral/penile pain or 'itchiness' should have a urethral swab culture for bacteria, including gonorrhea, as well as for chlamydia. We have found it useful to also culture for mycoplasma, another etiological agent responsible for urethritis.

Other tests

Cytological examination of the urine

Urinary frequency, dysuria and even bladder and penile pain can be associated with carcinoma in situ of the lower urinary tract. All patients with these constellations of symptoms should have a cytological examination of the urine to rule out atypical or malignant cells.

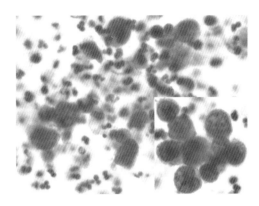

Urine cytology. The background image shows abnormal transitional cells in an inflammatory background while the inset shows these cells at higher power. The large size of the cells, high nuclear to cytoplasmic ratio, irregular nuclear contour and coarse chromatin pattern all indicate that the cells are malignant and consistent with transitional cell carcinoma. Both images are Papanicolaou ('pap') stain, background ×200, inset ×400.

Prostate specific antigen

Prostate specific antigen or PSA screening for prostate cancer has become almost standard in men over 50 and even younger. How does prostatitis

EVALUATION OF THE PROSTATITIS PATIENT
OTHER TESTS
Cytological examination of the urine
Prostate specific antigen

affect PSA testing? Certainly acute bacterial prostatitis can cause significant rises in PSA levels, as high as 50–100 ng/ml in some patients. The data concerning elevations of PSA in patients with chronic prostatitis syndrome are much more confusing. While some studies would indicate a modest elevation in PSA in prostatitis patients compared with normal asymptomatic patients, this has not been a universal finding. At this time, the author strongly advocates that PSA testing should be performed in patients presenting with chronic prostatitis symptoms, if the physician would be screening for prostate cancer anyway or if prostatic irregularity is noted on DRE. If the PSA is elevated and bacteria or inflammation are noted in prostate specific specimens, a trial of appropriate antibiotic therapy (likely a fluoroquinolone) and perhaps an anti-inflammatory agent for 4–6 weeks is reasonable before repeating the PSA. In most cases the physician should consider an elevated PSA in these men as they would any other elevated PSA in a screening population.

What about elevated PSA levels in men with Category IV asymptomatic inflammatory prostatitis? These patients are entirely asymptomatic as far as prostatitis symptoms are concerned but if looked for, may have white blood cells in their expressed prostatic secretion. At least one study has indicated that it would be appropriate to assess the leukocyte status of prostate specific specimens in patients with mildly elevated PSAs and then treat with appropriate antibiotic therapy before repeating the PSA. The author of this book feels that at this point, that approach is really not cost-effective and believes that it is prudent and safer to assess all asymptomatic men with elevated PSA in the same manner despite any findings in expressed prostatic secretion or post-prostatic massage urine. In fact, the author does not look for asymptomatic inflammatory prostatitis in his patients screened for prostate cancer, unless an initial biopsy is negative and an explanation is required for the elevated PSA.

Other tests

Cystoscopy

Is cystoscopy really necessary for every patient presenting with prostatitis? The answer is no, but the physician should be inclined to either do a cystoscopy or refer the patient to a urologist who can do a cystoscopy if the presentation is abnormal, hematuria is a presenting symptom, there is a history of genitourinary or perineal trauma, obstructive voiding is a major symptom and/or some form of surgical intervention is contemplated. In those cases, cystoscopy is not only suggested but is really mandatory to rule out correctable or serious lower urinary tract pathology.

Patients who present with suprapubic pain as their primary symptom should also be considered as possibly having interstitial cystitis. Cystoscopy under general anesthetic with hydrostatic bladder dilation may be helpful, not only in diagnosis but also in ameliorating symptoms.

Transrectal ultrasound

In the recent past, many felt that transrectal ultrasound could be used to diagnose prostatitis. Certainly it is one of the better tests to diagnose prostatic abscess and would be an important test to perform in a patient with acute bacterial prostatitis whose symptoms are not resolving with appropriate antibiotic therapy. However, in the chronic prostatitis syndromes, it is not usually very helpful. Small prostatic cysts, prostatic calcifications and stones are noted in many patients with and without prostatitis. However, as with cystoscopy, transrectal ultrasound is indicated in a number of patients. In patients with recurrent bacterial cystitis, it is important to know whether bacterial persistence is associated with prostatic calculi. In patients with abnormal DRE, transrectal ultrasound will help differentiate areas of focal calcification or possible areas that should be biopsied. In patients with large fluctuant masses on DRE, a prostate abscess or cyst should be ruled out by transrectal ultrasound. In patients in whom ejaculatory pain is the predominant symptom, ejaculatory duct cyst or obstruction or alternatively seminal vesicular abnormalities need to be ruled out.

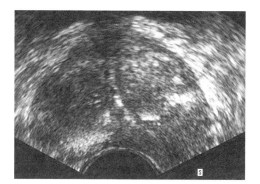

A transrectal ultrasound (TRUS) image of the prostate showing prostatic calcifications (central and peripheral), heterogeneity and echolucent zones in a patient with Category IIIA CP/CPPS

Abdominal/pelvic ultrasound, CAT scan, MRI

If the history or physical examination suggest any other possible pelvic or abdominal causes for the patient's symptoms, appropriate scans should be completed to rule out potentially important pathology.

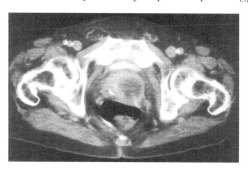

A CT scan showing the early abscess formation in the prostate of an acute bacterial prostatitis patient who was not responding appropriately to antibiotic therapy

Other tests

Urodynamics

Urodynamics are generally unhelpful in most patients presenting with chronic prostatitis but we have found that uroflowmetry and ultrasound residual urine determination are simple and effective screening tests. Patients who have a decreased maximum flow rate (<20 ml/s), increased residual urine (>50–100 ml) or in whom obstructive voiding is the predominant symptom and who do not respond to appropriate therapy (such as alpha-blocker therapy) should be further assessed with lower urinary tract urodynamic evaluation. Video-urodynamics with pressure-flow studies can be helpful in examining the bladder neck and evaluating voiding parameters. Patients with poor opening of the bladder neck (with bladder neck hyperplasia) and high voiding pressures may respond to transurethral incision of the bladder neck. This topic will be covered later in the treatment section of this book.

Recommended evaluation of patients with chronic prostatitis syndromes	
Mandatory	
History	
Physical examination, including digital rectal examination	
Lower urinary tract localization test (4-glass or 2-glass test)	
Recommended	
Symptom inventory or index (such as NIH-CPSI)	Flow rate
Urine cytology	Residual urine determination (by ultrasound)
Optional	
Semen analysis and culture	Transrectal ultrasound of the prostate
Urethral swab for culture	Pelvic CT scan
Pressure-flow studies	Prostate specific antigen (PSA)
Video-urodynamics (including flow-EMG studies)	

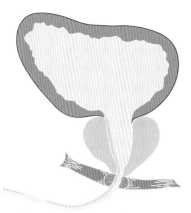

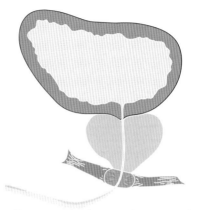

Detrusor–sphincter dyssynergia

Detrusor–bladder neck dyssynergia /
bladder neck hypertrophy

Flow rate

Detrusor
pressure

Abdominal
pressure

EMG tracing
(detrusor–
sphincter
dyssynergia

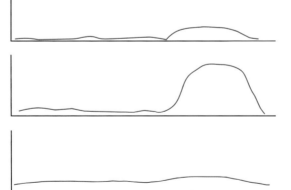

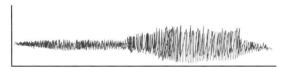

Typical
urodynamic
findings of a
CPPS patient
with
obstructive
voiding

Suggested reading

Aarnink RG, de la Rosette JJ. Imaging in prostatitis. In: Nickel JC (ed) Textbook of Prostatitis. Oxford: Isis Medical Media, 2000: 213–217.

Kohn IJ, Te AE, Kaplan SA. The role of urodynamics in evaluating patients with chronic prostatitis. In: Nickel JC (ed) Textbook of Prostatitis. Oxford: Isis Medical Media, 2000: 227–132.

Krieger JN, Nyberg LJ, Nickel JC. NIH consensus definition and classification of prostatitis. JAMA 1999; 282: 236–237.

Litwin MS, McNaughton-Collins M, Fowler FJJ et al. The National Institutes of Health chronic prostatitis symptom index: development and validation of a new outcome measure. J Urol 1999; 162: 369–375.

Ludwig M, Schroeder-Printzen I, Ludecke G, Weidner W. Comparison of expressed prostatic secretions with urine after prostatic massage – a means to diagnose chronic prostatitis/inflammatory chronic pelvic pain syndrome. Urology 2000; 55: 175–177.

Nickel JC. The Pre and Post Massage Test (PPMT): a simple screen for prostatitis. Tech Urol 1997; 3: 38–43.

CHAPTER 4
PRACTICAL THERAPEUTIC STRATEGIES FOR THE PROSTATITIS PATIENT: DEVELOPMENT OF A TREATMENT PLAN

Treatment for prostatitis has traditionally been empiric and not 'evidence-based'. The only exception to this general statement has been the evidence from clinical studies determining the efficacy of various antibiotics in the somewhat rare cases of acute and chronic bacterial prostatitis. For decades the only accepted outcome parameter was the eradication of bacteria, and therefore it is understandable that most prostatitis research was driven by the antimicrobial pharmaceutical business. Unfortunately, <5% of patients presenting with a prostatitis syndrome have a documented infection with a traditional uropathogen. For the majority of patients presenting with prostatitis, particularly the chronic prostatitis syndromes, reported therapeutic trials were sparse, small, and poorly designed. However, over the last several years, interesting pilot studies and well designed randomized placebo-controlled trials have been undertaken and reported, allowing the physician to practice a 'best evidence-based' approach to the treatment of prostatitis.

ACUTE BACTERIAL PROSTATITIS (NIH CATEGORY I): A SPECIAL CASE

Acute bacterial prostatitis is associated with a generalized infection of the prostate gland that is usually associated with acute cystitis, often with bacteremia and occasionally with septicemia. The objectives of treatment are simple.

Optimize urinary drainage

Many of these patients have obstructive voiding symptoms secondary to the inflamed, swollen prostate gland. If the patient is unable to empty his bladder, passing a small calibre urethral catheter may be all that is necessary. If there is a significant residual urine the catheter can be left in place. If the patient finds the catheter too uncomfortable or it is determined that it is too painful to pass the catheter, a temporary percutaneous suprapubic tube is indicated.

Eradicate the bacteria

After obtaining urine and blood cultures, the patient is started on intravenous, broad-spectrum antibiotic therapy. The best drugs are either a combination of penicillin (e.g. ampicillin) and an aminoglycoside (e.g. gentamicin), second or third generation cephalosporins or one of the fluoroquinolones. The patient is switched to a specific oral antibiotic, based on the culture and sensitivity data, as soon as the acute infection has settled down. The best oral antibiotics are either trimethoprim (or trimethoprim-sulfamethoxazole) or one the fluoroquinolones. The fluoroquinolone class of antibiotics appears to be superior. Antibiotics are continued for 2–4 weeks.

PRACTICAL THERAPEUTIC STRATEGIES: DEVELOPMENT OF A TREATMENT PLAN

ACUTE BACTERIAL PROSTATITIS (NIH CATEGORY I)

Optimize urinary drainage

Eradicate the bacteria

Supportive care

Close follow-up

Supportive care

General supportive care is given, including anti-pyrexic analgesics and intravenous fluid replacement as required.

Close follow-up

If patients do not respond in 36–48 hours, the physician should be suspicious that the patient may be developing a prostatic abscess. Prostatic abscesses are generally best drained transurethrally; however, transperineal and even transrectal approaches can be contemplated in some cases.

Acute bacterial prostatitis is rare, diagnosis is relatively simple, treatment is invariably successful. Few patients progress into a chronic prostatitis syndrome.

CHRONIC BACTERIAL PROSTATITIS (NIH CATEGORY II)

Patients with Category II chronic prostatitis present with either recurrent urinary tract infections (and are sometimes asymptomatic between these infections) or chronic prostatic and lower urinary tract symptoms indistinguishable from Category III chronic prostatitis/chronic pelvic pain syndrome patients.

Antibiotics

Once uropathogenic bacteria are localized to a prostate specific specimen (the specimen can be expressed prostatic secretion, post-prostatic massage urine or semen specimen), patients with either of these two presentations are treated primarily with antimicrobial therapy. On the basis of theoretical pharmacological principles, numerous animal studies in the 1970s and 1980s and a myriad of comparative antimicrobial clinical trials, two classes of antibiotics have justifiably emerged as optimal antibiotic therapy; trimethoprim-sulfamethoxazole and fluoroquinolones. Trimethoprim-sulfamethoxazole, one of the most studied antibiotics in prostatitis, owes its efficacy to trimethoprim rather than sulfamethoxazole. For that reason trimethoprim alone may be an appropriate choice and result in fewer side effects (by eliminating potential adverse events with sulfa medication). However, even with reasonable penetration into the prostate gland, long-term eradication of the offending bacteria occurs in only about 30–60% of cases. Significant improvement of symptoms occurs in about 40% of symptomatic patients. Fluoroquinolones would appear to have an advantage over trimethoprim, based on theoretical considerations, animal studies, bacterial sensitivities and prostatic tissue levels. Clinical studies appear to confirm improved efficacy of fluoroquinolones over trimethoprim or trimethoprim-sulfamethoxazole. The bacterial eradication rate is as high as 80–90% and the symptomatic improvement rate (in symptomatic chronic bacterial prostatitis patients) occurs in at least 50–60% of patients. The duration of therapy is controversial and various authors' and experts' suggestions have ranged from 4 to 12 weeks. In the rare patient in whom a uropathogenic bacterium is cultured in a prostate specific specimen, the physician should err on the side of too much antibiotic rather than too little.

What does the physician do when he finally encounters a patient with a confirmed chronic bacterial prostatitis, administers appropriate antibiotic therapy for a reasonable duration and then discovers that either the bacterial infection recurs or the patient's symptoms do not abate? For these patients, the physician must have a therapeutic plan in mind. Is it justified to continue antibiotics? If the patient had a symptomatic response while on the antibiotics, further antibiotic prescription can be justified. Is it justified to change the class of antibiotic? Certainly, if the patient was on trimethoprim-sulfamethoxazole, it would be appropriate to switch the patient to a quinolone antibiotic. Is it justified to switch from one fluoroquinolone to another fluoroquinolone? Studies have shown that ciprofloxacin has greater efficacy in eradicating bacteria than norfloxacin. Although studies would appear to indicate that ciprofloxacin, ofloxacin, levofloxacin and the other quinolone antibiotics are equally efficacious, comparative studies have not really been done and the anecdotal experience of many urologists suggests that some patients respond better to one antibiotic than another. There is some theoretical, anecdotal and even some clinical trial experience showing that adding tetracycline (doxycycline) or a macrolide (azithromycin, clarithromycin) may be of benefit. In some patients, who have a clinical response (reduction of symptoms) that recurs when antibiotics are discontinued, low-dose long-term suppressive therapy may be indicated. In patients who have frequent recurrent lower urinary tract infections, secondary to a bacterial nidus within the prostate gland that cannot be eradicated with a long duration of full-dose antibiotic therapy, low-dose prophylactic long-term therapy may be indicated.

Prostate massage

A number of investigators have advocated the combination of prostatic massage and antibiotic therapy. Theoretically, prostatic massage drains obstructed prostatic ducts, improving prostatic acinar and ductal prostatic secretion drainage and perhaps even temporarily improves local prostatic blood flow. Both of these considerations may improve antibiotic penetration into the prostate gland. The evidence remains anecdotal, but if the patient reports improvement of symptoms with prostate massage, then repetitive prostatic massage therapy should be considered.

Alpha-blockers

There is some clinical evidence that the addition of an alpha-blocker to antibiotics reduces the recurrence rate of patients with chronic bacterial prostatitis. The use of alpha-blockers and prostatic massage will be discussed more thoroughly in the next section (Category III CPPS).

Surgery

The consideration of surgical procedures to treat chronic bacterial prostatitis should not be taken lightly. There are very few studies reported in the literature (primarily just case reports) of employing

PRACTICAL THERAPEUTIC STRATEGIES: DEVELOPMENT OF A TREATMENT PLAN

CHRONIC BACTERIAL PROSTATITIS (NIH CATEGORY II

Antibiotics
Prostate massage
Alpha-blockers
Surgery

radical transurethral resection of the prostate and radical prostatectomy for patients with prostatitis. However, this author has significant experience (not only his own, but also patients referred to his prostatitis clinic) and would suggest to the reader that radical TURP or open total prostatectomy should only be entertained under the following scenarios.

1. Chronic bacterial prostatitis.
    (a) Recurrent lower urinary tract infection with the same organism.
    (b) The organism should be localized to the prostate between documented infections.
    (c) Prostatic calculi need to be radiologically documented.

2. Incidental diagnosis of prostate cancer.
    A prostate biopsy performed because of relatively high PSA, abnormal DRE or out of desperation (looking for positive bacterial cultures) may document prostate cancer.

Other than the two scenarios discussed above, this author would advise against radical surgery for patients presenting with Category II chronic bacterial prostatitis.

KEY POINTS

Modalities of treatment used for Category II chronic prostatitis

- Antibiotics

- Repetitive prostatic massage

- Alpha-blockers

- Surgery

CHRONIC PROSTATITIS/CHRONIC PELVIC PAIN SYNDROME (CATEGORY III)

The majority of patients who present to the clinician are diagnosed with this category of prostatitis. These patients complain of long-term pain, voiding disturbances, perhaps some sexual disturbances, all of which severely impact on their quality of life. They do not have documented infection of the lower urinary tract but may have demonstrable inflammation. Physicians must have a therapeutic plan, individualized to the patient's symptoms and clinical findings. Therapeutic suggestions and treatment algorithms presented in this section are based on relatively new data, recently published or presented, or studies just completed and not yet available to many physicians. Physicians and patients must have a realistic expectation of treatment goals. Patients' symptoms wax and wane and sometimes disappear completely (at least for a period of time). The physician's job is to ameliorate symptoms, decrease the impact the condition has on the patients' daily activities and subsequently improve the patients' quality of life. In most cases, this will not mean that the condition is cured and the patient must realize that the goal of therapy is amelioration of symptoms rather than a complete cure. We have found the use of the NIH Chronic Prostatitis Symptom Index to be invaluable in tracking this improvement. A 25% improvement in symptom score is a perceptible and even acceptable improvement in Category III CPPS. A 50% improvement in this score is an excellent response to therapy. These types of realistic therapeutic goals are achievable when employing the treatment algorithms described in this manual.

KEY POINT

■ Therapeutic goals: A 25% improvement in symptom score is a perceptible and even acceptable improvement rate in Category III CPPS. A 50% improvement in this score is an excellent response to therapy.

The treatment suggestions and algorithms presented in this section of the prostatitis manual should not be looked on as a rigid treatment plan. Many patients have already been treated with a number of the options presented, but perhaps they should be tried again, using a slightly different approach. If a patient has some amelioration of symptoms with a particular medication (particularly if it is a medication that requires long-term use) that medication is not discontinued but rather the next medication or treatment is added. This 'multi-modal' treatment plan is far more successful than starting and stopping multiple treatment options.

KEY POINT

■ Successful therapy for chronic prostatitis/chronic pelvic pain syndrome consists of a step-wise multi-modal approach to therapy; discontinuing therapies that don't work and continuing and adding therapies that provide benefit.

Conservative therapy

The patient diagnosed with CPPS will respond to a variety of conservative measures and it is important that the physician considers these before the patient and physician embark on the path of medical and surgical treatments. A discussion of the diagnosis of CPPS with an empathetic and knowledgeable physician is immediately empowering for the patient. 'He is not crazy.' The patient should be reassured that the condition does not usually progress over time and in fact tends to wax and wane and eventually improve over time (which may be months, years and occasionally decades). He should be counseled that although prostatitis is not associated with prostate cancer, he has the same risk as other men of developing this prostate problem and should be screened for prostate cancer as if he never had CPPS. The patient should avoid situations that induce stress and anxiety, as these factors can exacerbate symptoms of CPPS and cause serious flare-ups. Physical activities, such as bicycle riding, which may aggravate the situation, should be curtailed. Patients whose employment requires long periods of sitting, either in hard office chairs or poorly suspended trucks or heavy machinery, should modify the seat with a donut or air cushion. Gentle local heat application (hot sitz baths, heating pads, heated auto seats) can improve some of the local symptoms in many CPPS patients. Advice regarding diet is difficult, however, many patients find that avoiding caffeine (coffee, etc.), alcohol and spicy/acidic foods and drink helps control the symptoms. These conservative measures should be employed by the physician along with the therapies outlined below.

Conservative measures suggested for the amelioration of the symptoms of CP/CPPS
Diet avoid spicy foods, acidic foods/drinks, alcohol, caffeine
Lifestyle avoid stress and anxiety-provoking situations
Counseling develop coping and chronic pain management techniques
Work and play avoid repetitive perineal trauma (bicycle seats, hard chairs/seats, poor vehicle suspensions
Local heat therapy hot sitz baths, heating pad

Antibiotics

By definition, patients with Category III CPPS do not have a documented uropathogenic bacterial infection. Theoretically, therefore, they should not be treated with antibiotics. However, surveys over the last 10 years, carried out in many countries, have confirmed that the majority of patients (in fact almost all) presenting with chronic prostatitis are treated at least once with antibiotics. Why do physicians continue to treat chronic prostatitis with antibiotics even though in that particular patient no infection has been documented? It is because physicians have found that antibiotics ameliorate the symptoms in many patients with chronic prostatitis. A number of studies in the past have suggested that approximately 40% of patients treated with antibiotics show some clinical improvement. A recently published study by the Canadian Prostatitis Research Group documented this improvement using symptom scores (including the NIH-CPSI) as outcome parameters. Approximately 50% of patients, regardless of culture status (bacterial or non-bacterial) or leukocyte status (inflammatory or non-inflammatory CPPS) had significant clinical improvement when treated with quinolone antibiotics. This study indicated that a 4-week trial of antibiotic therapy could predict a patient's eventual response. If a patient has a perceptible clinical response following treatment with a quinolone antibiotic for 4 weeks, it would seem justified to continue that antibiotic therapy for a total of 8–12 weeks. If the patient has no response with the quinolone antibiotics, further antibiotic therapy would likely be futile. The fluoroquinolone class of antibiotics appears to be the optimal choice, although the possibility that some of these cases may be secondary to chlamydia or mycoplasma would seem to justify a trial of either a tetracycline (doxycycline) or a macrolide (azithromycin, clarithromycin).

Why should antibiotics benefit a patient who has no documented infection in the prostate gland or for that matter, the lower urinary tract? It might

65

be that the bacteria are present in the prostate gland in a small protected nidus. Our research team has shown that some patients with chronic bacterial prostatitis, appropriately treated with antibiotics, continue to have small focal aggregates of bacteria located deep in the prostate gland. These 'hibernating' bacteria are surrounded by a protective exopolysaccharide coating (called a glycocalyx). These small focal bacterial 'biofilms' deep within the prostate gland may continue to exert immunologic effects, particularly during flare-ups. Gram-positive bacteria such as coagulase-negative staphylococci, corynebacteria, or other micro-organisms such as chlamydia, mycoplasma or some other form of non-culturable cryptic micro-organism may also be responsible for the symptoms and may be suppressed by antibiotic therapy. Recently, antibiotics have been shown to have mild anti-inflammatory and even analgesic properties and these properties rather than the antimicrobial properties of antibiotics might be responsible for the mild amelioration of symptoms. The other possible explanation may be that the antibiotic therapy is nothing more than an excellent placebo and the observed amelioration of symptoms is only a pronounced placebo effect.

Physicians should watch out for the results of two major multi-center randomized controlled trials comparing antibiotic therapy to placebo in patients with Category III chronic pelvic pain syndrome. It is hoped that the results of these trials will be available in 2003.

KEY POINT

■ Antibiotic therapy appears to benefit some patients with chronic pelvic pain syndrome despite negative cultures for uropathogenic bacteria.

Doses of antibiotics typically used in patients with chronic prostatitis/chronic pelvic pain syndrome

Antibiotic	Dose
Trimethoprim-sulfamethoxazole (TMP-SMX – Septra, Bactrim)	800/160 mg twice/day
Norfloxacin (Noroxin)	400 mg twice/day
Ciprofloxacin (Cipro)	500 mg twice/day
Ofloxacin (Floxin)	300 mg twice/day
Lomefloxacin (Maxaquin)	400 mg once/day
Levofloxacin (Levaquin)	500 mg once/day
Gatifloxacin (Tequin)	400 mg once/day
Moxifloxacin (Avelox)	400 mg once/day
Doxycycline (Vibramycin)	100 mg twice/day
Erythromycin (Erythrocin)	500 mg four times/day
Azithromycin (Zithromax)	250–500 mg once/day
Clarithromycin (Biaxin)	500 mg twice/day

Chronic prostatitis/chronic pelvic pain syndrome (Category III)

Alpha-blockers

Alpha-blockers have become the most effective medical therapy to improve the lower urinary tract symptoms related to benign prostatic hyperplasia. Their action involves the relaxation of the prostatic capsular, prostatic stromal and bladder neck smooth muscle cells. This action also appears to improve the symptoms of some men presenting with a chronic prostatitis syndrome. The non-specific alpha-blocker, phenoxybenzamine, has been shown in small clinical trials to result in more improvement than placebo; however, patients could not tolerate the significant adverse effects of this non-specific alpha-blockade. A small study with a specific alpha-1-blocker, alfuzosin, suggested that it may be more efficacious than placebo; however, this study was too small and too short to make a definitive statement. A number of larger, but uncontrolled studies evaluating terazosin and doxazosin in this syndrome also suggested that alpha-1-blockade may reduce specific prostatitis symptoms in patients with CPPS. However, these studies were not

Alpha-blockers used in CP/CPPS	
Alpha-blocker	*Dose*
Terazosin (Hytrin)	5–10 mg/day
Doxazosin (Cardura)	4–8 mg/day
Tamsulosin (Flo-Max)	0.4–0.8 mg/day
Alfuzosin (Aatral-XL)	10 mg/day

randomized placebo-controlled. Despite the sparse evidence, alpha-blockers have become the second most common medical therapy employed by urologic specialists in this condition. The more specific alpha-1A-blockers, such as tamsulosin, appear to be the most popular therapeutic choice, however, there is no evidence from studies in the literature substantiating any claim that these more specific alpha-blockers are effective. Physicians should be on the look out for the results of a number of randomized controlled trials comparing alpha-blockers, including tamsulosin, to placebo which are presently underway. These results should be available in 2003.

Anti-inflammatories

It seems understandable that anti-inflammatory agents would be the third most common agent employed in the treatment of a presumed inflammatory condition. Up until recently, only one small study suggested any improvement when non-steroidal anti-inflammatory agents were employed. However, it is apparent that high doses of anti-inflammatory agents are required and this results either in intolerability or significant prevalence of adverse events. Cyclooxygenase-2 (COX-2) inhibitors allow for higher doses of medication with fewer side effects. A recent large, multi-center randomized placebo-controlled pilot study suggested that treatment with 50 mg of rofecoxib (a selective inhibitor of COX-2) for 6 weeks resulted in significant amelioration of pain and improvement of quality of life compared with placebo. Although a beneficial effect was noted at a dose of 25 mg/day of rofecoxib, the improvement was not significantly better than the placebo benefit. Further studies will be required to determine the exact role of long-term COX-2 inhibition in chronic prostatitis; however, the general use of anti-inflammatory agents, at least on a trial basis, appears to be justified. A number of investigators believe that the condition of interstitial cystitis, another inflammatory condition of the lower urinary tract associated with pelvic (and bladder) pain and irritative voiding symptoms which is a common diagnosis in women, is related to chronic prostatitis/chronic pelvic pain syndrome in men. A phase II pilot study evaluating pentosan polysulfate in men with CPPS noted amelioration of symptoms in a significant number following 6 months of therapy. A small single-center randomized placebo-controlled trial suggested mild improvement of symptoms compared with placebo. A recently completed multi-center randomized placebo-controlled trial also suggested that in some men with CPPS, 4 months of pentosan polysulfate results in more significant amelioration of symptoms than similar placebo therapy.

Anti-inflammatory agents commonly employed in CP/CPPS	
Anti-inflammatory agent	Dose
Ibuprofen (Motrin)	400–600 mg four-six times/day
Diclofenac (Voltarin)	25–50 mg three times/day
Indomethacin (Indocid)	25–50 mg three times/day
Rofecoxib (Vioxx)	25–50 mg/day
Celecoxib (Celebrex)	100–200 mg twice/day
Pentosan polysulfate (Elmiron)	100–300 mg three times/day

Hormone therapy

The development and function of the prostate gland is regulated by its hormonal milieu, primarily the balance between androgens and estrogens. It is felt by many investigators that in many cases the inflammatory process begins within the ducts and spills out into the ductal and peri-ductal tissues of the prostate gland. Anti-androgen therapy significantly reduces the ductal and acinar prostatic volume and may have an indirect effect on subsequent prostatic inflammation. A number of case series have suggested that there is a beneficial effect. A number of randomized controlled trials, two trials comparing finasteride to placebo and one comparing finasteride therapy to saw palmetto, have confirmed that patients (particularly those with inflammatory Category IIIA CPPS) experience a significant amelioration of their symptoms compared with baseline and that this affect appears to be modestly greater than that seen with either placebo or saw palmetto.

Hormonal agent commonly prescribed in CP/CPPS	
Hormonal agent	Dose
Finasteride (Proscar)	5 mg/day

Muscle relaxants

Patients with CP/CPPS appear to have an increased tone or even spasm of the skeletal and smooth muscle of the lower urinary tract, perineum and pelvic floor. This can sometimes be treated successfully with smooth muscle relaxants (see section on alpha-blockers) or skeletal muscle relaxants. Small studies have confirmed that some patients treated with diazepam or baclofen experience improvement in their generalized prostatitis symptoms.

Muscle relaxants commonly prescribed in CP/CPPS	
Relaxant	*Dose*
Diazepam (Valium)	5–10 mg/day
Baclofen (Lioresal)	5–20 mg three times/day
Cyclobenzaprine (Flexeril)	10 mg three times/day

Phytotherapeutic agents (plant extracts) and other supplements

The effects of three phytotherapeutic agents on the symptoms of prostatitis have been tested in small clinical trials. Bee pollen extract (Cernilton) therapy resulted in amelioration of symptoms in 50% of prostatitis patients treated in a clinical trial but this was not a randomized controlled trial. In a randomized controlled trial comparing saw palmetto to finasteride, after 6 months, patients treated with saw palmetto had no significant improvement compared to baseline (when they started therapy). A small short-term pilot study comparing the bioflavinoid, quercetin, to placebo indicated that patients treated with quercetin had a more significant clinical response than patients treated with placebo. Plant extracts have been shown to have a number of physiological effects, particularly in in-vitro studies, and it is not inconceivable that some of these compounds may have beneficial effect in

PRACTICAL THERAPEUTIC STRATEGIES: DEVELOPMENT OF A TREATMENT PLAN
CHRONIC PROSTATITIS/CHRONIC PELVIC PAIN SYNDROME (CATEGORY III)
Muscle relaxants
Phytotherapeutic agents (plant extracts) and other supplements
Other medical therapies

patients presenting with chronic prostatitis. Larger, multi-center randomized placebo-controlled trials are really needed to assess the effect of these plant extracts, but in the meantime there is some evidence that they may help and they certainly do not appear to cause any significant harm.

Although it appears that patients with prostate infections have lower zinc levels in the expressed prostatic fluid and in the prostate itself, zinc supplements have not yet been rigorously tested to determine if oral ingestion of zinc results in increased prostate zinc levels, reduced inflammation or improvement in symptoms.

Phytotherapies (plant extracts) and other supplements that have been suggested or tested in CP/CPPS	
Agent	Dose
Quercetin (Prosta-Q)	500 mg twice/day
Saw palmetto (Permixon)	160 mg twice/day
Bee pollen extract (Cernilton)	1 tablet three times/day
Zinc supplements	various doses recommended

Other medical therapies

Many other medical therapies have been advocated for the treatment of CP/CPPS and, while anecdotal reports and clinical experience appear to justify the claims of many of these therapies, either conflicting clinical data or no clinical data are available at this time. Initial clinical research with allopurinol suggested that the agent may alleviate the symptoms of CPPS, but subsequent data analysis and clinical experience has not corroborated the initial benefits. Amitriptyline is employed by physicians in many chronic pain conditions, such as interstitial cystitis and fibromyalgia, and while never confirmed in randomized placebo-controlled trials, appears to successfully ameliorate symptoms in many patients with CPPS. Similarly, gabapentin (Neurontin), particularly at high doses may reduce some of the neuropathic pain symptoms of some men with CPPS, but this perceived beneficial effect really needs to be confirmed in clinical trials. Patients themselves sometimes stumble on potentially effective therapy and the benefits are spread by word of mouth or even by the internet. Most of these therapies (the most popular at the time this manual was written appear to be variations of a broccoli-based treatment, various Chinese herbal remedies and urine alkalization) are usually innocuous, at least as effective as placebo therapy, and in some cases may actually be beneficial. Nevertheless, potentially harmful consequences should be reviewed with the patient by the physician.

Other medical therapies that have been recommended (but efficacy unproven) in CP/CPPS	
Therapy	*Dose*
Amitriptyline (Elavil)	10–100 mg/day
Allopurinol (Zyloprim)	300–600 mg/day
Gabapentin (Neurontin)	300–600 mg three times/day

Physical therapies

For most of the last century, prostate massage has been the therapy of choice (before antibiotics it was probably the only therapy available) for the treatment of chronic prostatitis. Theoretically, repetitive prostatic massage improved prostatic ductal drainage and perhaps influenced local blood flow. Anecdotally, many patients felt that they obtained significant relief (at least enough to repeatedly submit to this somewhat uncomfortable procedure). Following recommendations by the prostatitis gurus, Ed Meares and Tom Stamey, in the late 1960s, prostatic massages became a diagnostic and not a therapeutic procedure. However, recent interest, particularly among patient advocacy groups, has led to a resurgence of interest in this traditional therapy and its popularity is increasing. Anecdotal evidence has suggested that as many as one-third to two-thirds of patients may respond to repetitive prostatic massage. Based on clinical experience only, it has been suggested that bi-weekly or tri-weekly sessions be continued for 4–6 weeks before abandoning this therapeutic option.

On physical examination of patients with chronic pelvic pain syndrome, the physician often discovers discreet localized anatomic areas of

Physical therapies employed in the treatment of CP/CPPS	
Repetitive prostate massage	Biofeedback
Myofascial trigger point release therapy	Neuromodulation therapies
Relaxation exercises	Acupuncture

discomfort or pain. These areas in the perineum and pelvis can be the trigger point leading to the development of myofascial pain. Treatment of these trigger points can include heat therapy, physiotherapy massage, ischemic compression, stretching and progressive relaxation exercise, anesthetic injections, electroneuromodulation, yoga and acupuncture. Referral to a specialized physiotherapy clinic that would be willing to employ one of these innovative therapies can lead to significant improvement in symptoms and quality of life in motivated patients. A number of studies have indicated that biofeedback has the potential to improve symptoms in patients, particularly those whose pain and voiding symptoms may be secondary to some form of pseudodyssynergia during voiding or repetitive perineal muscle spasm.

Minimally invasive therapies

Almost every minimally invasive therapeutic procedure evaluated for benign prostatic hyperplasia has been advocated for the treatment of prostatitis. Transurethral balloon dilation, transurethral needle ablation of the prostate (TUNA), transurethral laser therapy and localized heat application employing transrectal hyperthermia or transurethral thermal therapy (TUMT) have all been tested in small, uncontrolled pilot studies. While the studies suggest that these minimally invasive therapies may improve the symptoms in some patients, the studies are too small, the patient population is ill-defined, the outcome parameters have not been validated and long-term results are unknown. These therapies cannot be generally advocated until more studies are available, except perhaps the heat therapies. There are a number of reasonably well designed, but small, randomized sham-controlled trials comparing heat therapy to sham therapy in the treatment of chronic prostatitis/chronic pelvic pain syndrome. Transrectal hyperthermia appears to be beneficial in patients with Category IIIB non-inflammatory CPPS while transurethral therapy appears to be most effective in patients with Category IIIA inflammatory CPPS. Transurethral microwave thermotherapy (TUMT) does have defined risks but may be considered as a last resort therapy in some desperate patients with inflammatory CPPS. It cannot be generally advocated until larger multi-center trials have been completed. Patients can benefit from localized heat therapy provided by hot sitz baths or heating pads. Many patients' complaints are very likely due to a chronic pelvic/perineal neuropathy and various invasive neuromodulatory therapies may be of benefit. We have not found peripheral afferent nerve stimulation (SANS) to be of any value, but others have reported that implanted nerve stimulators have reduced the pain and voiding symptoms of some CPPS patients. Proposed trials with these surgically implanted stimulators will confirm any benefits from this very aggressive modality of therapy.

Minimally invasive therapies evaluated in CP/CPPS	
Transurethral microwave thermotherapy (TUMT)	**Transurethral needle ablation of the prostate (TUNA)**
Transrectal hyperthermia	
	Prostatic laser therapies
Other heat therapies	
	Invasive neuromodulation (InterStim)
Transurethral balloon dilation	

Chronic prostatitis/chronic pelvic pain syndrome (Category III)

Surgery

Surgery does not have an important role in the treatment of most chronic prostatitis syndromes unless a specific indication is discovered during the evaluation of a patient. Severe obstructive phimosis, meatal stenosis, urethral stricture, documented seminal vesicle pathology, obstructed ejaculatory ducts, prostatic cysts, and bladder neck obstruction secondary to hypertrophy or contraction are all potential conditions that may be associated with refractory CPPS. These conditions are amenable to surgical treatment and this treatment usually results in improvement of voiding symptoms in many patients with subsequent improvement in the pain and discomfort associated with CPPS. Although some authors have advocated the use of radical TURP or even radical prostatectomy in patients with CPPS, this author, based on a number of patients referred to him with chronic prostatitis who have already had their prostate removed, would strongly advise against it. Our only indication at the present time for this type of radical surgery in patients with CPPS is associated incidental finding of localized prostate cancer.

Surgery for CP/CPPS	
Circumcision (phimosis causing obstruction, chronic balanitis or recurrent UTI)	Seminal vesicular surgery for documented seminal vesicular pathology
Urethral stricture surgery	Transurethral incision of the bladder neck
Drainage of prostatic abscesses, large prostatic cysts or obstructed ejaculatory ducts	Radical transurethral resection of the prostate
	Radical prostatectomy

ASYMPTOMATIC INFLAMMATORY PROSTATITIS (CATEGORY IV)

By definition patients diagnosed with Category IV AIP are asymptomatic. The diagnosis is made on pathological examination, TURP specimens, histologic examination of prostate biopsies, and microscopy of semen analysis in infertile men.

Antibiotic therapy (and perhaps anti-inflammatory therapy) may be indicated in some men with mildly elevated PSA, particularly if prostatic inflammation is noted on biopsies, and perhaps selected infertile men with leukospermia.

Therapy for Category IV asymptomatic inflammatory prostatitis (when indicated)	
Antibiotics	Anti-inflammatory agents

KEY POINT

■ Therapy for prostatitis was once empiric, but now can be based on 'best evidence' from clinical trials.

Suggested reading

Anderson RU. Treatment of prostatodynia (pelvic floor myalgia or chronic non-inflammatory pelvic pain syndrome). In: Nickel JC (ed) Textbook of Prostatitis. Oxford: Isis Medical Media, 1999: 357–364.

Bjerklund Johansen T, Gruneberg RN, Guibert J et al. The role of antibiotics in the treatment of chronic prostatitis: a consensus statement. Eur Urol 1998; 34: 457–466.

Evans DTP. Medical management of chronic nonbacterial prostatitis. In: Nickel JC (ed) Textbook of Prostatitis. Oxford: Isis Medical Media, 1999: 293–309.

Kirby RS. Surgical considerations in the management of prostatitis. In: Nickel JC (ed) Oxford: Isis Medical Media, 1999: 346–364.

McNaughton-Collins M, MacDonald R, Wilt TJ. Diagnosis and treatment of chronic abacterial prostatitis: a systematic review. Ann Intern Med 2000; 133: 367–381.

Naber KJ. Antibiotic treatment of chronic bacterial prostatitis. In: Nickel JC (ed) Textbook of Prostatitis. Oxford: Isis Medical Media, 1999: 283–292.

PRACTICAL STRATEGIES FOR THE TREATMENT OF PATIENTS WITH PROSTATITIS: A CLINICAL ALGORITHM

The Queen's University Department of Urology Prostatitis Research Clinic has been open for less than 10 years. We have thoroughly assessed and treated over 1000 patients; 750 patients have been entered into clinical trials. Based on our experience with these patients, our clinical trial experience, patients with prostatitis seen in our general urology clinics, and our comprehensive review of the world literature on the treatment of prostatitis, the author presents to the reader his strategic plan for patients with prostatitis. The plan is individualized, based on patients' previous treatments and response to those treatments, severity of symptoms, impact of the condition on the patient's quality of life and the NIH category based on the diagnostic algorithm described in Chapter 3.

CATEGORY I – ACUTE BACTERIAL PROSTATITIS

The patient is easily diagnosed and usually successfully treated with appropriate antibiotics, supportive therapy, and urinary drainage as outlined in Chapter 4. The rare patient who does not respond may have developed a prostate abscess which will require appropriate surgical drainage.

The author proposes a treatment algorithm for patients presenting with Category I bacterial prostatitis

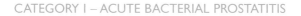

CATEGORY I

ACUTE BACTERIAL PROSTATITIS

CATHETERIZATION

INTRAVENOUS ANTIBIOTICS
(12-48 HOURS)

TRUS

TRANSURETHRAL DRAINAGE

ORAL ANTIBIOTICS
(3-4 WEEKS)

CURE

CATEGORY II/III – CHRONIC PROSTATITIS / CHRONIC PELVIC PAIN SYNDROME

The patient contract

Once a clinical diagnosis of CP/CPPS is made, we develop the physician–patient relationship with an unwritten and unsigned contract. We promise to investigate and to the best of our ability treat the patient's condition. We establish early on with the patient that we may not definitively identify the 'initiator' of the patient's condition but will attempt to define the status of the condition at the time of our evaluation. We then develop very realistic therapeutic goals with the patient; amelioration of symptoms rather than cure. The patient is made aware that we will be measuring his response to therapy employing the NIH-CPSI which measures the pain and voiding symptoms as well as the impact on quality of life, but we will also be using more informal, yet validated, subjective global assessments (the patient gives us a subjective estimate of the degree of improvement or not).

The investigation

All patients in our clinic undergo the diagnostic algorithm described in Chapter 3. All patients complete a demographic form which at minimum should outline his age, medical and surgical history, onset of prostatitis-like symptoms, previous investigations and treatments for the condition. All patients are asked to complete the Chronic Prostatitis Symptom Index at first visit. All patients undergo a focused physical examination. Because we are a research clinic we perform the 4-glass localization test (also culturing for chlamydia, mycoplasma and anaerobic bacteria), examine and culture semen and urethral swabs, and perform a uroflow as well as an ultrasound residual urine determination. This evaluation requires two visits and is not really required for most patients presenting to our regular urology clinic with the same diagnosis. The author suggests that physicians who are committed to their prostatitis patients collect at least

Category II/III – chronic prostatitis / chronic pelvic pain syndrome

a mid-stream urine followed by an initial stream urine specimen after DRE and prostate massage (the 2-glass test described in Chapter 3). The urine specimens will be sent for microscopy and culture. Further testing such as uroflowmetry, residual urine determination, cystoscopy, PSA, urodynamic evaluation, pelvic and abdominal radiologic evaluation, etc. would depend on individual circumstances of that particular patient.

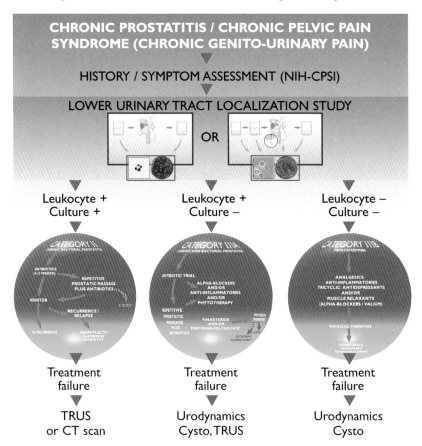

Based on this evaluation the patient should be categorized as NIH category II, IIIA or IIIB.

The patient with Category II chronic bacterial prostatitis

Patients with Category II chronic prostatitis are treated with a minimum of 8 (and usually 12) weeks of fluoroquinolone antibiotic. If the patient

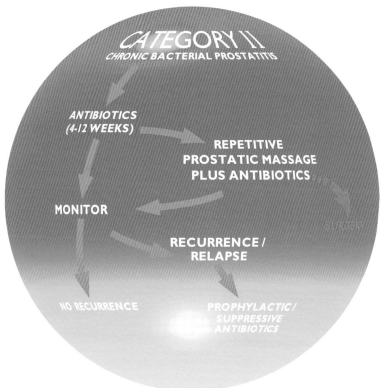

The author proposes a treatment algorithm for patients presenting with Category II chronic bacterial prostatitis

complains of any obstructive voiding symptoms, has a maximum flow rate of less than 20 cc/sec, residual urine of over 50 cc or is over the age of 50, we add an alpha-blocker (titrated to maximum tolerable dose). If the patient responds, the antibiotics are stopped at 12 weeks and the alpha-blockers continued for a minimum of 6 months. If the patient does not respond, we suggest the addition of repetitive prostate massage (two times per week for several minutes each time). In patients who have a relapse (microbiological relapse or a clinical relapse) the patient is kept on suppressive or prophylactic low-dose long-term antibiotic therapy.

The patient with Category III chronic pelvic pain syndrome

All patients are instructed regarding a patient-initiated and physician-directed conservative therapeutic plan. This includes diet modification (we suggest reduction of caffeine, spicy foods and alcohol), reduction of any physical initiating factors (i.e. bicycle riding, long car drives), local heat therapy (heating pads, heated car seats, hot baths), development of coping skills (based on education and realistic expectation of goals of therapy) and avoidance of stress and anxiety precipitators.

All patients diagnosed with category III CPPS are treated with an initial trial of at least 4 weeks of a quinolone antibiotic. Almost all patients referred to our prostatitis clinic have already been treated with antibiotics so for these patients we do not restart them unless it has been years since they have tried. Some patients referred to our primary care general urology clinics have not yet been treated with antibiotics and it is in these patients that we expect the best response to an antibiotic trial. If response is obtained, the antibiotic will be continued for a further 4-8 weeks. Patients who have urethral symptoms (discharge, urethral discomfort or dysuria) will be considered for a short 3-week course of tetracycline or a macrolide antibiotic (either concurrently or sequentially). Patients who have obstructive voiding symptoms, a maximum flow rate of less than 20 cc/sec, a residual urine of greater than 50 cc of urine or are over the age of 50 will also be treated with alpha-blockade, titrated to the maximum tolerable dose. Patients in whom pain is the major symptom will be treated with an anti-inflammatory agent. We tend to use a high

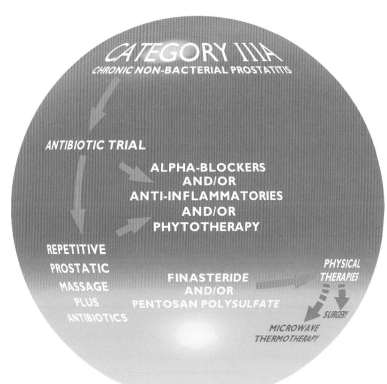

The author proposes a treatment algorithm for patients presenting with Category IIIA chronic pelvic pain syndrome

dose COX-2 inhibitor for 4-6 weeks. If response is obtained, the COX-2 inhibitor dose is reduced to a usual maintenance dose. Patients who are found on physical examination to have anal sphincter or perineal spasm are considered for skeletal muscle relaxants, either diazepam or baclofen. Patients who have completed antibiotic therapy and who have not had a significant resolution of symptoms, are started on a phytotherapeutic agent. In our clinic we tend to use quercetin. Our second line medical therapies for CPPS include finasteride and pentosan polysulfate. Patients, who are older than 40, have enlarged 'boggy' (soft) prostate glands in whom an excessive amount of EPS showing excessive leukocytosis can be expressed on prostatic massage are considered for a 6-month trial of finasteride. Patients in whom frequency, urgency and suprapubic discomfort are dominant symptoms, will be considered for a 6-month trial of pentosan polysulfate.

Depending on the type, location, chronicity and severity of the pain experienced by the patient, a referral to an anesthesia pain clinic is initiated. Our anesthetists use multiple approaches for relief of the chronic pain including tricyclic anti-depressants (amitriptyline), neuromodulators (gabapentin or Neurontin) controlled narcotic analgesia, trigger point injection (with a combination of local anesthetic and steroids), specific nerve blocks and in rare cases continuous epidural anesthesia. None of these approaches has ever been subjected to rigorous clinical trials; however, it has been our experience that many patients do achieve some relief of pain.

Medical therapy, as described above, does not always alleviate the symptoms of chronic prostatitis to the point where the patient is happy with the response. These patients undergo either physician-directed physical therapy (repetitive prostate massage) or are referred to our physiotherapy clinics. We have had reasonably good experience with biofeedback, acupuncture, pelvic floor massage and trigger point release therapy.

Patients with a definite indication for surgery (urethral stricture disease or bladder neck obstruction documented on video urodynamics) will be

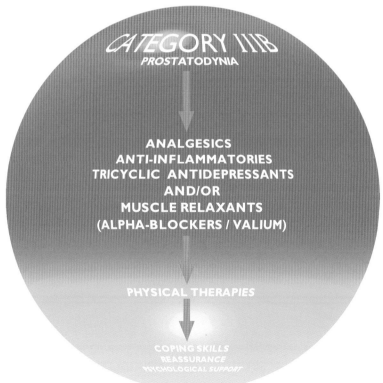

The author proposes a treatment algorithm for patients presenting with Category IIIB chronic pelvic pain syndrome

The patient with Category III chronic pelvic pain syndrome

offered definitive surgery while occasional patients with category IIIA CPPS will be offered, once they are appraised of the risks and benefits of the procedure, transurethral microwave thermal therapy. We do not advocate radical TURP or total prostatectomy in patients with CPPS unless there is a specific indication such as incidentally picked up prostate cancer.

KEY POINT

■ The key to successful amelioration of symptoms in CP/CPPS patients depends on an empathetic, interested and knowledgeable physician who is willing to proceed with a rational diagnostic plan and is able to formulate a 'best evidence-based' therapeutic strategy.

CATEGORY IV – ASYMPTOMATIC INFLAMMATORY PROSTATITIS

These patients are not referred to our Prostatitis Research Clinic, but we do see many such men in our general urology population. We do tend to treat infertile men who have associated leukospermia with antibiotics, usually a fluoroquinolone, but also a tetracycline or macrolide in patients with associated history or symptoms of urethritis. Except for dramatic rises in PSA in patients with Category I acute bacterial prostatitis, we are reluctant to attribute PSA elevations to chronic prostate inflammation unless the patient is symptomatic or else a previous biopsy documented histopathological evidence of prostate inflammation. In these patients, we feel that a 4-week trial of a quinolone antibiotic (we sometimes add an anti-inflammatory agent as well) may be appropriate before repeating the PSA and making a decision regarding prostate biopsy (either initial or repeat biopsy).

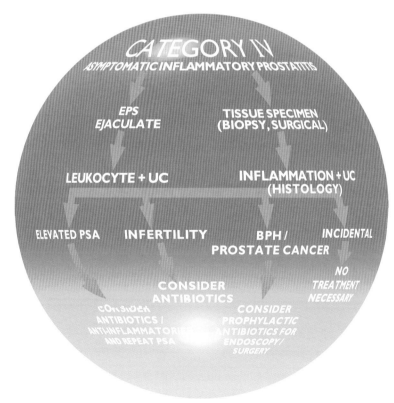

The author proposes a treatment algorithm for patients presenting with Category IV asymptomatic inflammatory prostatitis

Suggested reading

Nickel JC. Prostatitis: Evolving management strategies. Urol Clin North Am 1999; 26: 743-751.

Nickel JC. Prostatitis. In: Gillenwater, Grayhack, Howards, Mitchell (eds) Adult and Pediatric Urology. Philadelphia: WB Saunders, 2001.

Nickel JC. Prostatitis and related conditions. In: Walsh P et al (eds) Campbell's Urology, 8th edn. Philadelphia: WB Saunders, 2002.

CHAPTER 6

THE FUTURE FOR PROSTATITIS MANAGEMENT: A LIGHT AT THE END OF THE TUNNEL

More progress has been made in our understanding of the prostatitis syndromes and in developing evidence-based management programs for prostatitis patients in the last 5 years than in the last 50 years.

ETIOLOGY

Although we are still unsure of the etiology and pathogenesis of the condition in the majority of patients presenting to our clinic, considerable basic science and clinical research work is illuminating possible mechanisms. We understand now that this condition, actually a syndrome, encompasses a wide spectrum of related medical conditions. We know that the syndrome begins via stimulation from a wide variety of potential initiators and that the condition progresses through either an inflammatory or neuropathic (and sometimes both) pathway until the end stage, particularly for the chronic patient, is a patient with a chronic pelvic floor/perineal neuropathy. Future research holds the key to unlocking the exact mechanisms involved in the pain, voiding and sexual dysfunction associated with chronic prostatitis. Once this door is unlocked, specific mechanistic treatment plans will likely result in improved therapeutic results and perhaps even significant cure rates for chronic prostatitis.

DIAGNOSIS

We have defined the patient presenting to us with prostatitis. All patients are not immediately identified as having a 'prostate' problem and we realize that this condition is primarily a pelvic, pelvic floor and/or perineal problem. We have identified the major domains of the prostatitis experience; the pain/discomfort, voiding symptoms, sexual dysfunction and particularly the impact on quality of life. From this work we have developed a validated symptom score which can be used to assess the severity of disease, and follow therapeutic progress over time and which can be used as an outcome parameter in comparative clinical trials. We have 0 our diagnostic algorithm so it can be simple, cost-effective and attractive to the practicing physician.

TREATMENT

We have changed the focus of our treatment research from antibiotic therapy in the small percentage of patients presenting with chronic bacterial prostatitis to potentially effective innovative therapies for the vast majority of patients presenting to our clinic. The Prostatitis Foundation (www.prostatitis.org) has become a patient empowering organization that provides important educational and interactive resources for patients as well as physicians. Such patient advocacy groups have been invaluable in pressuring government granting agencies into funding prostatitis research endeavors. This influx of peer reviewed money encouraged the opening of many dedicated prostatitis research centers across North America (and even worldwide). An accepted definition and classification system and a validated outcome index have resulted in significant interest in the medical condition by pharmaceutical industries and equipment manufacturers. Companies with a potential product can now identify a large target population of potential customers and this realization of potential profit (as it did in benign prostatic hyperplasia) will result in an influx of research money and the initiation of many important clinical treatment trials. In fact, that has already been happening. Large multi-center trials are just being completed or are underway assessing the potential efficacy of antibiotics, alpha-blockers, finasteride, pentosan polysulfate, COX-2 inhibitors, immune suppressors and a number of minimally invasive surgical and neuromodulatory therapies. Other pilot studies presently underway will likely lead to further large multi-center randomized placebo-controlled trials. The results of these studies, many of which have been recently published or presented, allow the physician to practice a 'best evidence-based' treatment plan. This will improve therapy of our patients and result in less confusion and frustration among the medical profession in dealing with this enigmatic condition.

THE EVOLVING FIELD OF PROSTATITIS MANAGEMENT

The field of prostatitis research is evolving at a rapid pace. The etiologic, diagnostic and particularly the treatment considerations outlined in this manual are dynamic. Diagnostic tests and treatment strategies suggested in the manual will undergo change, some minor and some perhaps radical, as new information and data from basic science and clinical trials become available. Prostatitis research is at an exciting watershed. The benefits will spill over to physicians managing this urologic condition and particularly to patients who suffer from one of the prostatitis syndromes.

Suggested reading

Nickel JC. Prostatitis: perspectives for the 21st century. In Nickel JC (ed) Textbook of Prostatitis. Oxford: Isis Medical Media, 1999: 367-368.

Nickel JC. Prostatitis: Lessons from the 20th Century. BJU International 2000; 85: 179-185.

Nickel JC. Prostatitis: The Last Frontier. World Journal of Surgery 2000; 24: 1197-1199.

CHAPTER 7
BIBLIOGRAPHY

The explanations and suggestions regarding etiology, pathogenesis, diagnosis, and treatment of the prostatitis syndromes are based in part on a comprehensive review of the following literature. The opinions and interpretations of the data presented in these papers and studies are those of the author. The reader may want to know more details about the studies mentioned in the manual. This bibliography represents, in the author's opinion, a compendium of the best research done in the field of prostatitis over the last century.

Aarnink RG, de la Rosette JJ. Imaging in prostatitis. In: Nickel JC (ed) Textbook of Prostatitis. Oxford: Isis Medical Media, 2000: 213–217.

Abdelatif OM, Chandler FW, McGuire BSJ. *Chlamydia trachomatis* in chronic abacterial prostatitis: demonstration by colorimetric in situ hybridization. Hum Pathol 1991; 22: 41–44.

Alexander RB, Trissel D. Chronic prostatitis: results of an Internet survey. Urology 1996; 48: 568–574.

Alexander RB, Brady F, Ponniah S. Autoimmune prostatitis: evidence of T cell reactivity with normal prostatic proteins. Urology 1997; 50: 893–899.

Alexander RB, Ponniah S, Hasday J, Hebel JR. Elevated levels of proinflammatory cytokines in the semen of patients with chronic prostatitis/chronic pelvic pain syndrome. Urology 1998; 52: 744–749.

Anderson RU. Treatment of prostatodynia (pelvic floor myalgia or chronic non-inflammatory pelvic pain syndrome). In: Nickel JC (ed) Textbook of Prostatitis. Oxford: Isis Medical Media, 1999: 357–364.

Anderson RU, Fair WR. Physical and chemical determinations of prostatic secretion in benign hyperplasia, prostatitis and adenocarcinoma. Invest Urol 1976; 14: 137–140.

Anderson RU, Weller C. Prostatic secretion leukocyte studies in non-bacterial prostatitis (prostatosis). J Urol 1979; 121: 292–294.

Andreu A, Stapleton AE, Fennell C et al. Urovirulence determinene in *Escherichia coli* strains causing prostatitis. J Infect Dis 1997; 176: 464–469.

Attah E. Non-specific inflammatory lesions of the prostate: spectrum and patterns. Int Surg 1975; 60: 158–162.

Baert L, Leonard A. Chronic bacterial prostatitis: 10 years of experience with local antibiotics. J Urol 1988; 140: 755–757.

Baert L, Leonard A, D'Hoedt M, Vandeursen R. Seminal vesiculography in chronic bacterial prostatitis. J Urol 1986; 136: 844–845.

Barbalias GA. Prostatodynia or painful male urethral syndrome? Urology 1990; 36: 146–153.

Barbalias GA, Meares EM, Sant GR. Prostatodynia: clinical and urodynamic characteristics. J Urol 1983; 130: 514–517.

Barbalias GA, Nikiforidis G, Liatsikos EN. Alpha-blockers for the treatment of chronic prostatitis in combination with antibiotics. J Urol 1998; 159: 883–887.

Barnes RW, Hadley HL, O'Donoghue EPN. Transurethral resection of the prostate for chronic bacterial prostatitis. Prostate 1982; 3: 215–219.

Bates CP, Arnold EP, Griffiths DJ. The nature of the abnormality in bladder neck obstruction. Br J Urol 1975; 47: 651–656.

Baumueller A, Madsen PO. Experimental bacterial prostatitis in dogs. Urol Res 1977; 5: 211–213.

Becopoulos T, Georgoulias D, Constantinides C, Stathakis H, Kosmidis J. Acute prostatitis: which antibiotic to use first. J Chemother 1990; 2: 244–246.

Benson PJ, Smith CS. Cytomegalovirus prostatitis. Urology 1992; 40: 165–167.

Berger RE, Kessler D, Holmes KK. Etiology and manifestations of epididymitis in young men: correlations with sexual orientation. J Infect Dis 1987; 155: 1341–1343.

Berger RE, Krieger JN, Kessler D et al. Case-control study of men with suspected chronic idiopathic prostatitis. J Urol 1989; 141: 328–331.

Berger RE, Krieger JN, Rothman I, Muller CH, Hillier SL. Bacteria in the prostate tissue of men with idiopathic prostatic inflammation. J Urol 1997; 157: 863–865.

Berger RE, Miller JE, Rothman I, Krieger JN, Muller CH. Bladder petechiae after cystoscopy and hydrodistension in men diagnosed with prostate pain. J Urol 1998; 159: 83–85.

Berghuis JP, Heiman JR, Rothman I, Berger RE. Psychological and physical factors involved in chronic idiopathic prostatitis. J Psychosom Res 1996; 41: 313–325.

Bergman B. On the relevance of gram-positive bacteria in prostatitis. Infection 1994; 22 (Suppl 1): 22.

Bergman B, Wedren H, Holm SE. Staphylococcus saprophyticus in males with symptoms of chronic prostatitis. Urology 1989; 34: 241–245.

Bjerklund Johansen T, Gruneberg RN, Guibert J et al. The role of antibiotics in the treatment of chronic prostatitis: a consensus statement. Eur Urol 1998; 34: 457–466.

Blacklock NJ. Anatomical factors in prostatitis. Br J Urol 1974; 46: 47–54.

Blacklock NJ. Morphological and functional factors in prostatitis and its complications. Proc R Soc Med 1975; 68: 505–508.

Blacklock NJ. Urodynamic and psychometric observations and their implication in the management of prostatodynia. In: Weidner W, Brunner H, Krause W, Rothague CF (eds) Therapy of Prostatitis. Munich: Zuckswerdt Verlag, 1986: 201.

Blacklock NJ. The anatomy of the prostate: relationship with prostatic infection. Infection 1991; 19: S111–S114.

Blacklock NJ, Beavis JP. The response of prostatic fluid pH in inflammation. Br J Urol 1978; 46: 537–542.

Bourne CW, Frishette WA. Prostatic fluid analysis in prostatitis. J Urol 1967; 97: 140–144.

Bowers JE, Thomas GB. The clinical significance of abnormal prostatic secretions. J Urol 1958; 79: 976–982.

Boyle P, Keech M, Nonis A et al. The Urepik study: a cross-sectional survey of benign prostatic hyperplasia, urinary incontinence and male erectile dysfunction, prostatitis and interstitial cystitis in the UK, France, the Netherlands and Korea. J Epidemiol Biostat 1998; 3: 179–187.

Brahler E, Wurz J, Unger U et al. The "Giessen Prostatitis Symptom Score" (GSS): standardization of the questionnaire and prevalence of symptoms (abstract). J Urol 1997; 157 (Suppl 4): 239.

Bruce AW, Reid G. Prostatitis associated with Chlamydia trachomatis in 6 patients. J Urol 1989; 142: 1006–1007.

Bruce AW, Chadwick P, Willet WS et al. The role of chlamydia in genitourinary disease. J Urol 1981; 126: 625–629.

Buck AC, Rees RWM, Ebeling L. Treatment of chronic prostatitis and prostatodynia with pollen extract. Br J Urol 1989; 64: 496–499.

Campbell MF. Principles of urology: an introductory text to the diseases of the urogenital tract. Philadelphia: WB Saunders, 1957: 311–314.

Campbell TB, Kaufman L, Cook JL. Aspergillosis of the prostate associated with an indwelling bladder catheter: case report and review. Clin Infect Dis 1992; 14: 942–944.

Canale D, Scaricabarozzi I, Giorgi P. Use of a novel non-steroid anti-inflammatory drug, nimesulide, in the treatment of abacterial prostatovesiculitis. Andrologia 1993; 25: 163–166.

Canale D, Turchi P, Girogi PM, Scaricabarozzi I, Menchini-Fabris EF. Treatment of abacterial prostato-vasculitis with nimesulide. Drugs 1993; 46: 147–150.

Carson CC, McGraw VD, Zwadyk P. Bacterial prostatitis caused by Staphylococcus saprophyticus. Urology 1982; 19: 576–578

Chen KT, Schijj JJ. Coccidioidomycosis of the prostate. Urology 1985; 25: 82–84.

Chiang PH, Sai EM, Chiang CP. Pilot study of transurethral needle ablation (TUNA) in treatment of non bacterial prostatitis. J Endourol 1997; 11: 367–370.

Clemens JQ, Nadler RB, Schaeffer AJ, Bushman W. Biofeedback, pelvic floor re-education and bladder training for chronic pelvic pain syndrome in males. J Urol 2000; 163 (Suppl): 26 (abstract 114).

Cooper HG, MacLean JT. Chronic prostatitis associated with nonspecific urethritis. Can Med Assoc J 1946; 54: 136–144.

Correll I, Agace W, Klemm P et al. Type-1 fimbrial expression enhances *Escherichia coli* virulence for the urinary tract. Proc Natl Acad Sci USA 1996; 93: 9827–9832.

Cotran RS, Kumar V, Robbins SL. In: Robbins SL (ed) Robbins' Pathologic Basis of Disease, 6th edn. Philadelphia: WB Saunders, 1999: 1025–1027.

Dajani AM, O'Flynn JD. Prostatic abscess: a report of 25 cases. Br J Urol 1968; 40: 729–736.

Dalton DL. Elevated serum PSA due to acute bacterial prostatitis. Urology 1989; 33: 465.

Davis BE, Weigel JW. Adenocarcinoma of the prostate discovered in 2 young patients following total prostatovesiculectomy for refractory prostatitis. J Urol 1990; 144: 744–745.

de la Rosette JJ, Hubregtse MR, Karthaus HF, Debruyne FM. Results of a questionnaire among Dutch urologists and general practitioners concerning diagnostics and treatment of patients with prostatitis syndromes. Eur Urol 1992; 22: 14–19.

de la Rosette JJ, Karthaus HF, Debruyne FM. Ultrasonographic findings in patients with nonbacterial prostatitis. Urol Int 1992; 48: 323–326.

de la Rosette JJ, Karthaus HF, van Kerrebroeck PE, de Boo T, Debruyne FM. Research in 'prostatitis syndromes': the use of alfuzosin (a new alpha 1-receptor-blocking agent) in patients mainly presenting with micturition complaints of an irritative nature and confirmed urodynamic abnormalities. Eur Urol 1992; 22: 222–227.

de la Rosette JJ, Hubregtse MR, Meuleman EJ, Stolk-Engelaar MV, Debruyne FM. Diagnosis and treatment of 409 patients with prostatitis syndromes. Urology 1993; 41: 301–307.

de la Rosette JJ, Ruijgrok MC, Jeuken JM, Karthaus HF, Debruyne FM. Personality variables involved in chronic prostatitis. Urology 1993; 42: 654–662.

de la Rosette JJ, Giesen RJ, Huynen AL et al. Automated analysis and interpretation of transrectal ultrasonography images in patients with prostatitis. Eur Urol 1995; 27: 47–53.

Dik P, Lock TM, Schrier BP et al. Transurethral marsupialization of a medial prostatic cyst in patients with prostatitis-like symptoms. J Urol 1996; 155: 1301–1304.

Dilworth, JP, Neal DE Jr, Fussell EN, Roberts JA. Experimental prostatitis in non-human primates: I. Bacterial adherence in the urethra. Prostate 1990; 17: 227–231.

Di Trapani D, Pavone C, Serretta V et al. Chronic prostatitis and prostatodynia: ultrasonographic alterations of the prostate, bladder neck, seminal vesicles and periprostatic venous plexus. Eur Urol 1988; 15: 230–234.

Doble A. The diagnosis, aetiology and pathogenesis of chronic non-bacterial prostatitis. In: Nickel JC (ed) Textbook of Prostatitis. Oxford: Isis Medical Media, 1999: 123–127.

Doble A, Carter SS. Ultrasonographic findings in prostatitis. Urol Clin North Am 1989; 16: 763–772.

Doble A, Thomas BJ, Furr PM et al. A search for infectious agents in chronic abacterial prostatitis using ultrasound guided biopsy. Br J Urol 1989; 64: 297–301.

Doble A, Thomas BJ, Walker MM, Harris JR, Witherow RO, Taylor-Robinson D. The role of *Chlamydia trachomatis* in chronic abacterial prostatitis: a study using ultrasound guided biopsy. J Urol 1989; 141: 332–333.

Doble A, Walker MM, Harris JR, Taylor-Robinson D, Witherow RO. Intraprostatic antibody deposition in chronic abacterial prostatitis. Br J Urol 1990; 65: 598–605.

Doble A, Harris JR, Taylor-Robinson D. Prostatodynia and herpes simplex virus infection. Urology 1991; 38: 247–248.

Domingue GJ. Cryptic bacterial infection in chronic prostatitis: diagnostic and therapeutic implications. Curr Opin Urol 1998; 8: 45–49.

Domingue GJ, Human LG, Hellstrom WJ. Hidden microorganisms in "abacterial" prostatitis/prostatodynia. J Urol 1997; 157: 243.

Donadio AC, Gagliano H, Remedi MM, Nowotny E, Depiante-Depaoli M. Time-course study of cellular immune response and testosterone metabolism in an autoimmune model for chronic prostatic inflammation. J Urol 1998; 160: 1546–1550.

Dowling KJ, Roberts JA, Kaack MB. P-fimbriated *E. coli* urinary tract infection: a clinical correlation. South Med J 1987; 80: 1533–1536.

Drabick JJ, Gambel JM, Mackey JF. Prostatodynia in United Nations Peace Keeping Forces in Haiti. Milit Med 1997; 162: 380–383.

Drach GW. Problems in diagnosis of bacterial prostatitis: gram-negative, gram-positive and mixed infections. J Urol 1974; 111: 630–636.

Drach GW. Trimethoprim–sulfamethoxazole therapy of chronic bacterial prostatitis. J Urol 1974; 111: 637–639.

Drach GW. Chronic bacterial prostatitis: problems in diagnosis and therapy. Urol 1986; 27 (Suppl): 26–30.

Drach GW, Fair WR, Meares EM, Stamey TA. Classification of benign diseases associated with prostatic pain: prostatitis or prostatodynia? J Urol 1978; 120: 266.

Drummand AC. Trichomonas infestation of the prostate gland. Am J Surg 1936; 31: 98–103.

Dunnick NR, Ford K, Osborne D et al. Seminal vesiculography: limited value in vesiculitis. Urology 1982; 20: 454–457.

Dunzendorfer U, Kruschwitz K, Letzel H. Effects of phenoxybenzamine on clinical picture, laboratory test results and spermatogram in chronic abacterial prostatitis. Therapiewoche 1983; 33: 4694–4705.

Egan KJ, Krieger JL. Psychological problems in chronic prostatitis patients with pain. Clin J Pain 1994; 10: 218–226.

Egan KJ, Krieger JL. Chronic abacterial prostatitis – a urological chronic pain syndrome? Pain 1997; 69: 213–218.

Evans DTP. Medical management of chronic nonbacterial prostatitis. In: Nickel JC (ed) Textbook of Prostatitis. Oxford: Isis Medical Media, 1999: 293–309.

Eykyn S, Bultitude MI, Mayo ME, Lloyd-Davies RW. Prostatic calculi as a source of recurrent bacteruria in the male. Br J Urol 1974; 46: 527–532.

Eyre RC, Aaronson AG, Weinstein BJ. Palisading granulomas of the prostate associated with prior prostatic surgery. J Urol 1986; 136: 121–122.

Fair WR, Cordonnier JJ. The pH of prostatic fluid: a re-appraisal and therapeutic implications. J Urol 1978; 120: 695–698.

Fair WR, Couch J, Wehner N. Prostatic antibacterial factor. Identity and significance. Urology 1976; 7: 169–177.

Farman F. Classification of prostatitis. J Urol 1930; 23: 113–117.

Fish DN, Danziger LH. Antimicrobial treatment for chronic prostatitis as a means of defining the role of *Ureaplasma urealyticum*. Urol Int 1993; 51: 129–132.

Fowler JEJ, Mariano M. Difficulties in quantitating the contribution of urethral bacteria to prostatic fluid and seminal fluid cultures. J Urol 1984; 132: 471–473.

Fowler JEJ, Mariano M. Longitudinal studies of prostatic fluid immunoglobulin in men with bacterial prostatitis. J Urol 1984; 131: 363–369.

Frazier HA, Spalding TH, Paulson DF. Total prostatoseminal vesiculectomy in the treatment of debilitating perineal pain. J Urol 1992; 148: 409–411.

Galley Hf, Nelson SJ, Dubbels AM, Webster NR. Effect of ciprofloxacin on the accumulation of interleukin-6, interleukin-8, and nitrite from a human endothelial cell model of sepsis. Crit Care Med 1997; 25: 1392–1395.

Gardner W Jr, Culberson D, Bennett B. *Trichomonas vaginalis* in the prostate gland. Arch Pathol Lab Med 1996; 110: 430–432.

Gasser TC, Larsen EH, Dorflinger T, Madsen PO. The influence of various body fluids and pH on *E. coli* MIC of quinolone derivatives. In: Weidner W (ed) Therapy of Prostatitis: Experimental and Clinical Data. Munich: Zuckschwerdt, 1986: 50–53.

George NJ, Reading C. Sympathetic nervous system and dysfunction of the lower urinary tract. Clin Sci 1986; 70 (Suppl 14): 69–76.

Giannopoulos A, Koratzanis G, Giamareloos-Bourboulis J et al. Pharmacokinetics of clarithromycin in the prostate: implications for the treatment of chronic abacterial prostatitis. J Urol 2001; 165: 97–99.

Golz R, Mendling W. Candidosis of the prostate: a rare form of endomycosis. Mycoses 1991; 34: 381–384.

Gonder MJ. Prostatitis. Lancet 1963; 83: 305–306.

Granados EA, Riley G, Salvador J, Vincent J. Prostatic abscess: diagnosis and treatment. J Urol 1992; 148: 80–82.

Gumus B, Sengila Z, Solak M et al. Evaluation of non-invasive clinical samples in chronic chlamydial prostatitis by using in situ hybridization. Scand J Urol Nephrol 1997; 31: 449–451.

Hanno P. Therapeutic principles of anti-microbial therapy and new anti-microbial agents. Urol Clin North Am 1986; 13: 577–590.

Harada K, Tanahashi Y, Igari D et al. Clinical evaluation of inside echo patterns in gray scale prostatic echography. J Urol 1980; 124: 216–220.

Hasui Y, Marutsuka K, Asada Y et al. Relationship between serum prostate specific antigen and histological prostatitis in patients with benign prostatic hyperplasia. Prostate 1994; 25: 91–96.

Heidler H. Clinical effects of ciprofloxacin: clinical results in chronic bacterial prostatitis. In: Lode H (ed) Ciprofloxacin in Clinical Practice: New Light on Established and Emerging Uses. Stuttgart: Zuckschwerdt, 1990: 53–56.

Hellstrom W, Schmidt RA, Lue TF, Tanagho EA. Neuromuscular dysfunction in nonbacterial prostatitis. Urology 1987; 30: 183–188.

Henline RB. Prostatitis and seminal vesiculitis: acute and chronic. JAMA 1943; November 6: 608–615.

Hennenfent BR, Feleciano AE Jr. Thrice weekly prostatic drainage, microbial diagnosis, and anti-microbial therapy for bacterial prostatitis, non-bacterial prostatitis, prostatodynia and benign prostatic hyperplasia as practiced in the Philippines. J Urol 1997; 157 (Suppl): 239A.

Hennenfent BR, Feliciano AE Jr. Changes in white blood cell counts in men undergoing thrice-weekly prostatic massage, microbial diagnosis and antimicrobial therapy for genitourinary complaints. Br J Urol 1998; 81: 370–376.

Hitchens AP, Brown CP. The bacteriology of chronic prostatitis. Am J Public Health 1913; 3: 884–891.

Hochreiter WW, Duncan JL, Schaeffer AJ. Evaluation of the bacterial flora of the prostate using a 16 SrRNA gene based chain reaction. J Urol 2000; 163: 127–130.

Hochreiter WW, Nadler RB, Koch AE et al. Diagnostic value of serial cytokine changes in expressed prostatic secretions. J Urol 2000; 163 (Suppl): 24.

Holm M, Meyhoff HH. Chronic prostatic pain; a new treatment option with finasteride? Scand J Urol Nephrol 1996; 31: 213–215.

Huggins C, Masina MH, Eichelberger L, Wharton JD. Quantitative studies of the prostatic secretion. I. Characteristics of the normal secretion, the influence of the thyroid, suprarenal and testes extirpation and androgen substitution on the prostatic outlet. J Exp Med 1939; 70: 543–556.

Indudhara R, Singh SK, Vaidynanthan S, Banerjee CK. Isolated invasive candidal prostatitis. Urol Int 1992; 48: 362–364.

Isaacs JT. *Ureaplasma urealyticum* in the urogenital tract of patients with chronic prostatitis or related symptomatology. Br J Urol 1993; 72: 918–921.

Jacobsen JD, Kvist E. Prostatic abscess. A review of literature and a presentation of 5 cases. Scand J Urol Nephrol 1993; 27: 281–284.

Jameson RM. Sexual activity and the variations of the white cell content of the prostatic secretion. Invest Urol 1967; 5: 297–302.

Jarvi K, Mittleman M. Prostatitis in infertility. In: Nickel JC (ed) Textbook of Prostatitis. Oxford: Isis Medical Media, 1999: 233–240.

Jimenez-Cruz JF, Martinez FM, Allona AA, De Rafael L, Navio-Nino S, Baquero MM. Prostatitis: are the gram-positive organisms pathogenic? Eur Urol 1984; 10: 311–314.

Jimenez-Cruz JF, Tormo FB, Gomez JG. Treatment of chronic prostatitis: intraprostatic antibiotic injections under echography control. J Urol 1988; 139: 967–970.

John H, Barghorn A, Funke G et al. Non-inflammatory chronic pelvic pain syndrome: immunological study in blood, ejaculate and prostate tissue. Eur Urol 2001; 39: 72–78.

Kaplan SA, Te AE, Jacobs BZ. Urodynamic evidence of vesical neck obstruction in men with misdiagnosed chronic nonbacterial prostatitis and the therapeutic role of endoscopic incision of the bladder neck. J Urol 1994; 152: 2063–2065.

Kaplan SA, Ikeguchie F, Santarosa RP et al. Etiology of voiding dysfunction in men less than 50 years of age. Urology 1996; 47: 836–839.

Kaplan SA, Santarosa RP, D'Alisera PM et al. Pseudodyssynergia (contraction of the external sphincter during voiding) misdiagnosed as chronic nonbacterial prostatitis and the role of biofeedback as a therapeutic option. J Urol 1997; 157: 2234–2237.

Kawamura N. Trichomoniasis of the prostate. Jpn J Clin Urol 1973; 27: 335.

Keay S, Zhang CO, Baldwin BR et al. Polymerase chain reaction amplification of bacterial 16s rRNA genes in prostate biopsies from men without chronic prostatitis. Urology 1999; 53: 487–491.

Keltikangas-Jarvinen L, Ruokalainen J, Lethonen T. Personality pathology underlying chronic prostatitis. Psychother Psychosomat 1982; 37: 87–95.

Kennelly MJ, Oesterling JE. Conservative management of a seminal vesicle abscess. J Urol 1989; 141: 1432–1433.

Kirby RS. Surgical considerations in the management of prostatitis. In: Nickel JC (ed) Textbook of Prostatitis. Oxford: Isis Medical Media, 1999: 346–364.

Kirby RS, Lowe D, Bultitude MI, Shuttleworth KED. Intraprostatic urinary reflux: an aetiological factor in abacterial prostatitis. Br J Urol 1982; 54: 729–731.

Kobayashi TK, Araki H. Immunocytochemical detection of chlamydial antigen in both the urethral scraping and prostatic aspirate in a case of abacterial prostatitis. Acta Cytol 1988; 32: 270–272.

Koff W. Clinical trial comparing lomefloxacin and ofloxacin in the treatment of chronic bacterial prostatitis. Rev Bras Med 1996; 53: 88–91.

Kohn IJ, Te AE, Kaplan SA. The role of urodynamics in evaluating patients with chronic prostatitis. In: Nickel JC (ed) Textbook of Prostatitis. Oxford: Isis Medical Media, 1999: 227–132.

Kohnen PW, Drach GW. Patterns of inflammation in prostatic hyperplasia: a histologic and bacteriologic study. J Urol 1979; 121: 755–760.

Koroku M, Kumamoto Y, Hirose T. A study on the role of Chlamydia trachomatis in chronic prostatitis – analysis of anti-Chlamydia trachomatis specific IgA in expressed prostate secretion by western-blotting method. Kansenshogaku Zasshi 1995; 69: 426–437.

Krieger JN. Urologic aspects of trichomoniasis. Invest Urol 1981; 18: 411–417.

Krieger JN, Egan KJ. Comprehensive evaluation and treatment of 75 men referred to chronic prostatitis clinic. Urology 1991; 38: 11–19.

Krieger JN, Egan KJ, Ross SO, Jacobs R, Berger RE. Chronic pelvic pains represent the most prominent urogenital symptoms of "chronic prostatitis". Urology 1996; 48: 715–721.

Krieger JN, Riley DE, Roberts MC, Berger RE. Prokaryotic DNA sequences in patients with chronic idiopathic prostatitis. J Clin Microbiol 1996; 34: 3120–3128.

Krieger JN, Nyberg LJ, Nickel JC. NIH consensus definition and classification of prostatitis. JAMA 1999; 282: 236–237.

Krieger JN, Jacobs R, Ross SO. Detecting urethral and prostatic inflammation in patients with chronic prostatitis. Urol 2000; 55: 186–192.

Krieger JN, Jacobs R, Ross SO. Does the chronic prostatitis/pelvic pain syndrome differ from non-bacterial prostatitis and prostatodynia? J Urol 2000; 164: 1554–1558.

Kuberski T. Trichomonas vaginalis associated with nongonococcal urethritis and prostatitis. Sex Transm Dis 1980; 7: 135–136.

Kumon H. Detection of a local prostatic immune response to bacterial prostatitis. Infection 1992; 20: 5236–5238.

Kumon H. Immunological aspects of prostatitis. In: Nickel JC (ed) Textbook of Prostatitis. Oxford: Isis Medical Media, 1999: 157–164.

Kuroda K, Sawamura Y, Tajima M et al. Detection of Chlamydia trachomatis in urethra of patients with urogenital infection. Hinyokika Kiyo 1989; 35: 453–456.

Lafontaine PD, Middleman BR, Graham SD Jr, Sanders WH. Incidence of granulomatous prostatitis and acid-fast bacilli after intravesicular BCG therapy. Urology 1997; 49: 363–366.

Lang MD, Nickel JC, Olson ME, Howard SR, Ceri H. Rat model of experimentally induced abacterial prostatitis. Prostate 2000; 45: 201–206.

Lapatin WB, Martynik M, Hickey DP, Vivas C, Hakala TR. Retrograde transurethral balloon dilation of prostate: innovative management of abacterial chronic prostatitis and prostatodynia. Urology 1990; 36: 508–510.

Lee JC, Yang CC, Kromm BG, Berger RE. Neurophysiologic testing in chronic pelvic pain syndrome: a pilot study. Urology 2001; 58: 246–250.

Lepor H, Sypher D, Machi G, Derus J. Randomized double-blind study comparing the effectiveness of balloon dilation of the prostate and cystoscopy in the treatment of symptomatic benign prostatic hyperplasia. J Urol 1992; 147: 639–644.

Leskinen M, Lukkarinen O, Marttilla T. Effects of finasteride in patients with inflammatory chronic pelvic pain syndrome: a double-blind, placebo controlled, pilot study. Urology 1999; 53: 502–505.

Littrup PJ, Lee F, McLeary RD et al. Transrectal US of the seminal vesicles and ejaculatory ducts; clinical correlation. Radiology 1988; 168: 625–628.

Litwin MS, McNaughton-Collins M, Fowler FJJ et al. The National Institutes of Health chronic prostatitis symptom index: development and validation of a new outcome measure. J Urol 1999; 162: 369–375.

Lomberg H, Cedergren B, Leffler H et al. Influence of blood groups on the bio-availability of receptors for attachment of uropathogenic *Escherichia coli.* Infect Immun 1986; 51: 919–926.

Lopez-Plaza I, Bostwick DG. Prostatitis. In: Bostwick DG (ed) Pathology of the Prostate. New York: Churchill Livingstone, 1990: 15–30.

Lowe FC, Fagelman E. Phytotherapeutic agents in the treatment of chronic prostatitis. In: Nickel JC (ed) Textbook of Prostatitis. Oxford: Isis Medical Media, 1999: 329–331.

Lowentritt JE, Kawahara K, Human LG, Hellstrom WJ, Domingue GJ. Bacterial infection in prostatodynia. J Urol 1995; 154: 1378–1381.

Ludwig M, Weidner W, Schroeder-Printzen I, Zimmermann O, Ringert RH. Transrectal prostatic sonography as a useful diagnostic means for patients with chronic prostatitis or prostatodynia. Br J Urol 1994; 73: 664–668.

Ludwig M, Schroeder-Printzen I, Ludecke G, Weidner W. Comparison of expressed prostatic secretions with urine after prostatic massage – a means to diagnose chronic prostatitis/inflammatory chronic pelvic pain syndrome. Urology 2000; 55: 175–177.

Ludwig M, Steltz C, Huwe P et al. Immunocytological analysis of leukocyte sub-populations in urine specimens before and after prostatic massage. Eur Urol 2001; 39: 277–282.

McClinton S, Miller ID, Eremin O. An immunohistochemical characterization of the inflammatory cell infiltrate in benign and malignant prostatic disease. Br J Cancer 1990; 61: 400–401.

McGuire EJ, Lytton B. Bacterial prostatitis: treatment with trimethoprim-sulfamethoxazole. Urology 1976; 7. 499–500.

McNaughton-Collins M, O'Leary M. Prostatitis symptom scores. In: Nickel JC (ed) Textbook of Prostatitis. Oxford: Isis Medical Media, 1999: 187–196.

McNaughton-Collins M, Stafford RS, O'Leary MP, Barry MJ. How common is prostatitis? A national survey of physician visits. J Urol 1998; 159: 1224–1228.

McNaughton-Collins M, Stafford RS, O'Leary MP, Barry MJ. Distinguishing chronic prostatitis and benign prostatic hyperplasia symptoms: results of a national survey of physician visits. Urology 1999; 53: 921–925.

McNaughton-Collins M, Fowler FJ, Elliott DB, Albertsen PC, Barry MJ. Diagnosing and treating chronic prostatitis: do urologists use the four-glass test. Urology 2000; 55: 403–407.

McNaughton-Collins M, MacDonald R, Wilt TJ. Diagnosis and treatment of chronic abacterial prostatitis: a systematic review. Ann Intern Med 2000; 133: 367–381.

McNaughton-Collins M, O'Leary MP, Litwin MS et al. Quality of life is impaired in men with chronic prostatitis: results from the NIH Cohort study. J Urol 2000; 163 (Suppl): 23 (abstract 98).

McNeal JE. Regional morphology and pathology of the prostate. Am J Clin Pathol 1968; 49: 347–357.

Madsen PO, Baumueller A, Hoyme U. Experimental models for determination of antimicrobials in prostatic tissue, interstitial fluid and secretion. Scand J Infect Dis Suppl 1978; 145–150.

Madsen PO, Drescher P, Gasser TC. Basis for anti-bacterial treatment of prostatitis: experimental and clinical pharmacokinetic studies and models. In: Weidner W, Madsen PO, Schiefer HG (eds) Prostatitis: Etiopathology, Diagnosis and Therapy. Berlin: Springer, 1994: 110–122.

Mardh PA, Colleen S. Chlamydia in chronic prostatitis. Scand J Urol Nephrol 1972; 9: 8–16.

Mardh PA, Colleen S. Search for uro-genital tract infections in patients with symptoms of prostatitis. Studies on aerobic and strictly anaerobic bacteria, mycoplasmas, fungi, trichomonads and viruses. Scand J Urol Nephrol 1975; 9: 8–16.

Mardh PA, Ripa KT, Colleen S, Treharne JD, Darougar S. Role of *Chlamydia trachomatis* in non-acute prostatitis. Br J Vener Dis 1978; 54: 330–14.

Marmar JL, Praiss DE, Katz S et al. A protocol for evaluation of prostatitis. Urology 1980; 16: 261–265.

Mayo ME, Ross SO, Krieger JN. Few patients with "chronic prostatitis" have significant bladder outlet obstruction. Urology 1998; 52: 417–421.

Meares EM Jr. Observations on the activity of trimethoprim-sulfamethoxazole in the prostate. J Infect Dis 1973; 129 (Suppl): 679–685.

Meares EM Jr. Infection stones of prostate gland. Laboratory diagnosis and clinical management. Urology 1974; 4: 560–566.

Meares EM Jr. Long-term therapy of chronic bacterial prostatitis with trimethoprim-sulfamethoxazole. Can Med Assoc J 1975; 112 (Suppl): 22–25.

Meares EM Jr. Serum antibody titers in urethritis and chronic bacterial prostatitis. Urology 1977; 10: 305–309.

Meares EM Jr. Serum antibody titers in treatment with trimethoprim-sulfamethoxazole for chronic prostatitis. Urology 1978; 11: 141–146.

Meares EM Jr. Acute and chronic prostatitis: diagnosis and treatment. Infect Dis Clin North Am 1987; 1: 855–873.

Meares EM Jr. Acute and chronic prostatitis and prostatodynia. In: Fitzpatrick JM, Krane RJ (eds) The Prostate. Edinburgh: Churchill Livingstone, 1989: 62–75.

Meares EM Jr. Prostatitis and related disorders. In: Walsh PC, Retik AB, Vaughan ED, Wein AJ (eds) Campbell's Urology, 7th edn. Philadelphia: WB Saunders, 1998: 615–530.

Meares EM Jr, Stamey TA. Bacteriologic localization patterns in bacterial prostatitis and urethritis. Invest Urol 1968; 5: 492–518.

Mehik A, Hellstrom P, Lukkarinen O, Sarpola A, Alfthan O. Increased intraprostatic pressure in patients with chronic prostatitis. Urol Res 1999; 27: 277–279.

Mehik A, Hellstrom P, Lukkarinen O, Sarpola A, Jarvelin M. Epidemiology of prostatitis in Finnish men: a population-based cross-sectional study. BJUI 86: 443, 200.

Mehik A, Hellstrom P, Sarpola A et al. Fears, sexual disturbances and personality features in men with prostatitis: a population-based cross-sectional study in Finland. BJU International 2001: 88: 35–38.

Mehik A, Hellstrom P, Nickel JC et al. Chronic prostatitis/chronic pelvic pain syndrome can be characterized by prostatic tissue pressure measurements. J Urol 2002, 167: 137–140.

Mellan J, Raboch J, Kohlicek J. The problem of prostatic neurosis. Cesk Psychiatr 1973; 69: 112–117.

Mendlewich J, Schulman CC, De Schutter B, Wilmotte J. Chronic prostatitis: psychosomatic incidence. Psychother Psychosom 1971; 19: 118.

Mies C, Balogh K, Stadecker M. Palisading prostate granulomas following surgery. Am J Surg Pathol 1984; 8: 217–221.

Miller JL, Rothman I, Vavendam TG, Berger RE. Prostatodynia and interstitial cystitis: one and the same? Urology 1995; 45: 587–590.

Miyashita H, Troncoso P, Babaian RJ. BCG-induced granulomatous prostatitis: a comparative ultrasound and pathologic study. Urology 1992; 39: 364–367.

Mobley DE. Erythromycin plus sodium bicarbonate in chronic bacterial prostatitis. Urology 1974; 3: 60–62.

Mobley DE. Bacterial prostatitis: treatment with carbenicillin indanyl sodium. Invest Urol 1981;19: 31–33.

Moon TD. Questionnaire survey of urologists and primary care physicians' diagnostic and treatment practices for prostatitis. Urology 1997; 50: 543–547.

Moon TD. Immunology of chronic prostatitis: etiological and therapeutic considerations. Curr Opin Urol 1998; 8: 39–43.

Moon TD, Clegan S, Neal DE Jr. Prostate specific antigen and prostatitis II. PSA production and release kinetics in vitro. Prostate 1992; 20: 113–116.

Moon TD, Hagen L, Heisey DM. Urinary symptomatology in younger men. Urology 1997; 50: 700–703.

Muller CH, Berger RE, Mohr LE, Krieger JN. Comparison of microscopic methods for detecting inflammation in expressed prostatic secretions. J Urol 2001; 166: 2518–2524.

Murnaghan BF, Millard RJ. Urodynamic evaluation of bladder neck obstruction in chronic prostatitis. Br J Urol 1984; 56: 713–716.

Naber KJ. Antibiotic treatment of chronic bacterial prostatitis. In: Nickel JC (ed) Textbook of Prostatitis. Oxford: Isis Medical Media, 1999: 283–292.

Naber KG, Giamarellou H. Proposed study design in prostatitis. Infection 1994; 22: S59–S61.

Naber KJ, Madsen PO. Antibiotics: basic concepts. In: Nickel JC (ed) Textbook of Prostatitis. Oxford: Isis Medical Media, 1999: 83–94.

Nadler RB, Humphrey PA, Smith DS et al. Effect of inflammation and benign prostatic hyperplasia on elevated serum prostate specific antigen levels. J Urol 1995; 154: 407–413.

Nadler RB, Koch AE, Campbell PL et al. Interleukin IL-1beta and TNF-alpha in prostatic secretions are indicators in the evaluation of men with chronic prostatitis. J Urol 2000; 164 (in press).

Neal DE Jr. Treatment of acute prostatitis. In: Nickel JC (ed) Textbook of Prostatitis. Oxford: Isis Medical Media, 1999: 279–284.

Neal DE Jr, Moon TD. Use of terazosin in prostatodynia and validation of a symptom score questionnaire. Urology 1994; 43: 460–465.

Neal DE Jr, Dilworth JP, Kaack MB et al. Experimental prostatitis in non-human primates: II. Ascending acute prostatitis. Prostate 1990; 17: 233–239.

Neal DE Jr, Clejan S, Sarma D, Moon TD. Prostate specific antigen and prostatitis. I. Effect of prostatitis on serum PSA in the human and nonhuman primate. Prostate 1992; 20: 105–111.

Nickel AC. The bacteriology of chronic prostatitis and seminal vesiculitis and elective localization of the bacteria as isolated. J Urol 1930; 24: 343–357.

Nickel JC. Practical approach to the management of prostatitis. Tech Urol 1995; 1: 162–167.

Nickel JC. Rational management of nonbacterial prostatitis and prostatodynia. Curr Opin Urol 1996; 6: 53–58.

Nickel JC. The Pre and Post Massage Test (PPMT): a simple screen for prostatitis. Tech Urol 1997; 3: 38–43.

Nickel JC. The role of the animal model in the study of prostatitis. In: Bergan T (ed) Urinary Tract Infections. Basel: Karger, 1997: 89–97.

Nickel JC. Effective office management of chronic prostatitis. Urol Clin North Am 1998; 25: 677–684.

Nickel JC. Prostatitis: myths and realities. Urology 1998; 51: 362–366.

Nickel JC. Prostatitis: an historic perspective. In: Nickel JC (ed) Textbook of Prostatitis. Oxford: Isis Medical Media, 1999: 3–17.

Nickel JC. Prostatitis: evolving management strategies. Urol Clin North Am 1999; 26: 743–751.

Nickel JC. 5 alpha reductase therapy for chronic prostatitis. In: Nickel JC (ed) Textbook of Prostatitis. Oxford: Isis Medical Media, 1999: 333–337.

Nickel JC. Heat therapy for chronic prostatitis. In: Nickel JC (ed) Textbook of Prostatitis. Oxford: Isis Medical Media, 1999: 339–346.

Nickel JC. Prostatitis: perspectives for the 21st century. In: Nickel JC (ed) Textbook of Prostatitis. Oxford: Isis Medical Media, 1999: 367–368.

Nickel JC. Antibiotics for bacterial prostatitis. J Urol 2000; 163: 1407.

Nickel JC. Prostatitis: an infectious disease? Infect Urol 2000; 13: 31–38.

Nickel JC. Prostatitis: lessons from the 20th Century. BJU International 2000; 85: 179–185.

Nickel JC. Prostatitis syndromes: an update for urologic practice. Can J Urol 2000; 7: 1091–1098.

Nickel JC. Prostatitis: The Last Frontier. World J Surg 2000; 24: 1197–1199.

Nickel JC, Costerton JW. Coagulase-negative staphylococcus in chronic prostatitis. J Urol 1992; 147: 398–400.

Nickel JC, Costerton JW. Bacterial localization in antibiotic-refractory chronic bacterial prostatitis. Prostate 1993; 23: 107–114.

Nickel JC, MacLean RJL. Bacterial biofilms in urology. Infect Urol 1998; 11: 168–175.

Nickel JC, Sorensen R. Transurethral microwave thermotherapy for nonbacterial prostatitis: a randomized double-blind sham controlled study using new prostatitis specific assessment questionnaires. J Urol 1996; 155: 1950–1954.

Nickel JC, Weidner W. Chronic prostatitis: current concepts in antimicrobial therapy. Infect Urol 2000; 13: S22–S29.

Nickel JC, Bruce AW, Reid G. Pathogenesis, diagnosis and treatment of the prostatitis syndromes. In: Krane RJ, Siroky MB (eds) Clinical Urology. Philadelphia: JB Lippincott, 1994: 925.

Nickel JC, Costerton JW, McLean RJ, Olson M. Bacterial biofilms: influence on the pathogenesis, diagnosis and treatment of urinary tract infections. J Antimicrob Chemother 1994; 33: 31–41.

Nickel JC, Downey J, Clark J, Ceri H, Olson M. Antibiotic pharmacokinetics in the inflamed prostate. J Urol 1995; 153: 527–529.

Nickel JC, Siemens DR, Lundie MJ. Allopurinol for prostatitis: where is the evidence? Lancet 1996; 347: 1711–1712.

Nickel JC, Nigro M, Valiquette L et al. Diagnosis and treatment of prostatitis in Canada. Urology 1998; 52: 797–802.

Nickel JC, Siemens DR, Johnston B. Transurethral radiofrequency hot balloon thermal therapy in chronic nonbacterial prostatitis. Tech Urol 1998; 4: 128–130.

Nickel JC, Alexander R, Anderson R et al. Prostatitis unplugged: prostate massage revisited. Tech Urol 1999; 5: 1–7.

Nickel JC, Downey J, Feliciano AEJ, Hennenfent B. Repetitive prostatic massage therapy for chronic refractory prostatitis: the Philippine experience. Tech Urol 1999; 5: 146–151.

Nickel JC, Downey J, Young I, Boag A. Asymptomatic inflammation and/or infection in benign prostatic hyperplasia. Br J Urol 1999; 84: 976–981.

Nickel JC, Nyberg LM, Hennenfent M. Research guidelines for chronic prostatitis: consensus report from the first National Institutes of Health International Prostatitis Collaborative Network. Urology 1999; 54: 229–233.

Nickel JC, Johnston, Downey J et al. Pentosan polysulfate therapy for chronic nonbacterial prostatitis (chronic pelvic pain syndrome category IIIA): a prospective multicenter clinical trial. Urology 2000; 56: 413–417.

Nickel JC, Downey J, Hunter D, Clark J. Prevalance of prostatitis-like symptoms in a population based study employing the NIH-chronic prostatitis symptom index (NIH-CPSI). J Urol 2001; 165: 842.

Nickel JC, Downey J, Johnston B, Clark J and the Canadian Prostatitis Research Group. Predictors of patient response to antibiotic therapy for chronic prostatitis/chronic pelvic pain syndrome: a prospective multicenter clinical trial. J Urol 2001; 165: 1539–1544.

Nickel JC, Gittleman, Malek G et al. Effects of rofecoxib in patients with chronic nonbacterial prostatitis: a placebo controlled pilot study. J Urol 2001; 165 (Suppl): 27 (abstract 114).

Nickel JC, McNaughton-Collins M, Litwin SM. Use of a validated outcome measure for prostatitis. Journal of Clinical Outcomes Management 2001; 8: 30–37.

Nickel JC, True LD, Kreiger JN, Berger RE, Boag AH, Young I. Consensus development of a histopathological classification system for chronic prostatic inflammation. BJU International 2001; 87: 797–805.

Nickel JC, Siemens DR, Nickel KR, Downey J. The patient with chronic epididymitis: characterization of an enigmatic syndrome. J Urol 2002; 167: 1701–1704.

Nielsen ML, Justesen J. Studies on the pathology of prostatitis. A search for prostatic infections with obligate anaerobes in patients with chronic prostatitis and chronic urethritis. Scand J Urol Nephrol 1974; 8: 1–6.

Nilsson S, Johanisson G, Lycke E. Isolation of *C. trachomatis* from the urethra and prostatic fluid in men with signs and symptoms of acute urethritis. Acta Dermatol Venereol 1981; 61: 456–459.

Nishimura T. Prostatitis: especially concerning studies of leukocytosis in prostatic fluid and bacterial culture, and daily practice. Nippon Ika Daigaku Zasshi 1997; 64: 2–8.

Nishimura T, Terashima Y, Hattori T, Satoh M, Yoshida K, Akimoto M. Study of macrophages in prostatic fluid from nonbacterial prostatitis patients. V. Relation between activation of macrophages and stage of prostatitis. Urol Int 1991; 46: 15–17.

Novicki DE, Larson TR, Swanson SK. Interstitial cystitis in men. Urology 1998; 52: 621–624.

Oates RD, Stilmant MM, Freedlun MC, Siroky MB. Granulomous prostatitis following Bacillus Calmette-Guerin immunotherapy of bladder cancer. J Urol 1988; 140: 751–754.

O'Conor VJ. Therapeutic value of prostatic massage: with a discussion on prostatitis and the significance of proper rectal palpation of the prostate gland. Med Clin North Am 1936; 19: 1181–1185.

Ohkawa M, Yamaguchi K, Tokunaga S, Nakashima T, Fujita S. *Ureaplasma urealyticum* in the urogenital tract of patients with chronic prostatitis or related symptomatology. Br J Urol 1993; 72: 918–921.

Ohkawa M, Yamaguchi K, Tokunaga S, Nakashima T, Shoda R. Antimicrobial treatment for chronic prostatitis as a means of defining the role of *Ureaplasma urealyticum*. Urol Int 1993; 51: 129–132.

O'Leary M, Barry M, Fowler F. Hard measures of subjective outcomes: validating symptom indices in urology. J Urol 1992; 148: 1546–1548.

O'Leary MP, McNaughton-Collins M, Santanna J et al. Are there long term changes in symptoms over time in men with chronic prostatitis? An interim report from the Chronic Prostatitis Cohort (CPC) study. J Urol 2001; 165 (Suppl 5): 24 (abstract 100).

Oliveri RA, Sachs RM, Castl PG. Clinical experiences with geocillin in the treatment of bacterial prostatitis. Curr Ther Res 1979; 25: 415–421.

Orland SM, Hanno PM, Wein AJ. Prostatitis, prostatosis and prostatodynia. Urology 1985; 25: 439–459.

Osborn DE, George NJR, Rao PN. Prostatodynia – physiological characteristics and rational management with muscle relaxants. Br J Urol 1981; 156: 621–623.

O'Shaughnessy EJ, Parrinno PS, White JD. Chronic prostatitis – fact or fiction? JAMA 1956; Feb 18: 540–542.

Pai MG, Baht HS. Prostatic abscess. J Urol 1972; 108: 599–600.

Patel PS, Wilbur AC. Cystic seminal vesiculitis: CT demonstration. J Comput Assist Tomogr 1987; 11: 1103–1104.

Paulson DE, White RD. Trimethoprim-sulfamethoxazole and minocycline hydrochloride in the treatment of culture-proved bacterial prostatitis. J Urol 1978; 120: 184–185.

Peeling WB, Griffiths GJ. Imaging of the prostate by ultrasound. J Urol 1984; 132: 217–224.

Perachino M, Bozzo W, Vitali A, Puppo P, Ardoino S, Ferro MA. Does transurethral thermotherapy induce a long-term alpha blockade? Eur Urol 1993; 23: 299–301.

Persson BE, Ronquist G. Evidence for a mechanistic association between nonbacterial prostatitis and levels of urate and creatinine in expressed prostatic secretion. J Urol 1996; 155: 958–960.

Persson BE, Ronquist G, Ekblom M. Ameliorative effect of allopurinol on nonbacterial prostatitis: a parallel double-blind controlled study. J Urol 1996; 155: 961–964.

Pfau A. Bacterial prostatitis caused by *Staphylococcus saprophyticus*. Urology 1983; 21: 102–103.

Pfau A. The treatment of chronic bacterial prostatitis. Infection 1991; 19 (Suppl 3): 160–164.

Pfau A, Perlberg S, Shapira A. The pH of the prostatic fluid in health and disease: implications of treatment in chronic bacterial prostatitis. J Urol 1978; 119: 384–387.

Poletti F, Medici MC, Alinovi A, Menozzi MG, Sacchini P. Isolation of *Chlamydia trachomatis* from the prostatic cells in patients affected by nonacute abacterial prostatitis. J Urol 1985; 134: 691–693.

Potts JM. Prospective identification of National Institutes of Health Category IV prostatitis in men with elevated prostate specific antigen. J Urol 2000; 164: 1550–1553.

Pust RA, Ackenheil-Koppe HR, Gilbert P, Weidner W. Clinical efficacy of ofloxacin (Tarivid) in patients with chronic bacterial prostatitis: preliminary results. J Chemother 1989; 1 (Suppl 4): 469–471.

Ramiraz CT, Ruiz JA, Gomez AZ et al. A crystalographic study of prostatic calculi. J Urol 1980; 124: 840–843.

Ramirez RCH, Saavedra S, Fernandez MI et al. Bacteriology and microbiological complications in patients with chronic bacterial prostatitis (CBP) after using quinolones. 6th International Congress of Infectious Diseases, Prague, Czech Republic, April 1994, abstract 232.

Riedasch G, Mohring K, Ritz E. Antibody-coated bacteria in ejaculate in bacterial prostatitis. Urology 1984; 23: 252–255.

Riedasch G, Mohring K, Ritz E. Do antibody-coated bacteria prove bacterial prostatitis? Infection 1991; 19: S141–S143.

Riegel P, Ruimy R, De Briel D et al. *Corynebacterium seminale* sp.nov., a new species associated with genital infections in male patients. J Clin Microbiol 1995; 33: 2244–2249.

Riley DE, Berger RE, Miner DC, Krieger JN. Diverse and related 16S rRNA-encoding DNA sequences in prostate tissues of men with chronic prostatitis. J Clin Microbiol 1998; 36: 1646–1652.

Ritter JS, Lippow C. Pathological and bacteriological processes present in prostatitis and tissue reaction to therapy. J Urol 1938; 39: 111–117.

Roberts RO, Lieber MM, Bostwick DG, Jacobsen SJ. A review of clinical and pathological prostatitis syndromes. Urology 1997; 49: 809–821.

Roberts RO, Lieber MM, Rhodes T, Girman CJ, Bostwick DG, Jacobsen SJ. Prevalence of a physician-assigned diagnosis of prostatitis: the Olmsted County Study of Urinary Symptoms and Health Status Among Men. Urology 1998; 51: 578–584.

Roberts RO, Jacobson DJ, Lieber MM et al. Prevalence of prostatitis-like symptoms in community-dwelling men. J Urol 2001; 165 (Suppl 5): 24 (abstract 102).

Robertson C, Boyle P, Nonis A et al. International population-based study of urological conditions: the Urepik study. II. Comparative prostatitis data. J Urol 1999; 4 (Suppl): 32A.

Robertson C, Boyle P, Mazzetta C et al. The healthcare burden of prostatitis: the Urepik study. Eur Urol 2000; 37 (Suppl 2): 46.

Rovik J, Doehlin I. Prostatic abscess: imaging with transrectal ultrasound. Scand J Urol Nephrol 1989; 23: 307–308.

Rugendorff EW, Weidner W, Ebeling L. Results of treatment with pollen extract (Cernilton N) in chronic prostatitis and prostatodynia. Br J Urol 1993; 71: 433–438.

Ruggieri MR, Braverman AS, Filer-Marten S et al. Biochemical markers for inflammation and glands that contribute to the semen in chronic prostatitis patients. J Urol 2000; 163 (Suppl): 26.

Sahin A, Eiley D, Goldfischer ER et al. The in vitro bactericidal effect of microwave energy on bacteria that cause prostatitis. Urology 1998; 52: 411–415.

Sant GR, Kominski A. Interstitial cystitis in men is frequently misdiagnosed as non-bacterial prostatitis/prostatodynia. Abstracts of the NIDDK/NIH/ICA 1997 International Research Symposium on Interstitial Cystitis, October 30–31, Washington DC, 1997: 31.

Sant GR, Nickel JC. Interstitial cystitis in chronic prostatitis: the same syndrome? In: Nickel JC (ed) Textbook of Prostatitis. Oxford: Isis Medical Media, 1999: 169–176.

Sant GR, Heaney JA, Meares EM. "Radical" transurethral prostatic resection in the management of chronic bacterial prostatitis. J Urol 1984; 131 (Suppl): 184A.

Saw KC, Hartfal WG, Rowe RCG. Tuberculous prostatitis: nodularity may simulate malignancy. Br J Urol 1993; 72: 249–749.

Schaeffer AJ. Potential role of phase variation of type 1 pili in urinary tract infection and bacterial prostatitis. Infection 1991; 19: S144–S149.

Schaeffer AJ, Darras FS. The efficacy of norfloxacin in the treatment of chronic bacterial prostatitis refractory to trimethoprim-sulfamethoxazole and/or carbenicillin. J Urol 1990; 144: 690–693.

Schaeffer AJ, Wendel EF, Dunn JK, Grayhack JT. Prevalence and significance of prostatic inflammation. J Urol 1981; 125: 215–219.

Schappert S. National Ambulatory Medical Care Survey, 1991 Summary. Vital Health Stat [13] 1994; 116.

Schwarz J. Mycotic prostatitis. Urology 1982; 19: 1–5.

Serel TA, Kosar A, Osturk A et al. Treatment with neodymium: Yag laser in patients with chronic prostatitis: a preliminary report. Int Urol Nephrol 1997; 29: 53–58.

Sharer WC, Fair WR. The pharmacokinetics of antibiotic diffusion in chronic bacterial prostatitis. Prostate 1982; 3: 139–148.

Shaw TK, Watson GM, Barnes DG. Microwave hyperthermia in the treatment of chronic abacterial prostatitis and prostatodynia: results of a double-blind placebo controlled trial. J Urol 1993; 149 (Suppl): 405A.

Shortliffe LM, Wehner N. The characterization of bacterial and nonbacterial prostatitis by prostatic immunoglobulins. Medicine 1986; 65: 399–414.

Shortliffe LM, Wehner N, Stamey TA. The detection of a local prostatic immunologic response to bacterial prostatitis. J Urol 1981; 125: 509–515.

Shortliffe LM, Wehner N, Stamey TA. Use of a solid-phase radioimmunoassay and formalin-fixed whole bacterial antigen in the detection of antigen-specific immunoglobulin in prostatic fluid. J Clin Invest 1981; 67: 790–799.

Shortliffe LM, Elliott K, Sellers RG. Measurement of urinary antibodies to crude bacterial antigen in patients with chronic bacterial prostatitis. J Urol 1989; 141: 632–636.

Shortliffe LM, Sellers RG, Schachter J. The characterization of nonbacterial prostatitis: search for an etiology. J Urol 1992; 148: 1461–1466.

Shoskes DA, Moody JA. Prostatodynia. In: Nickel JC (ed) Textbook of Prostatitis. Oxford: Isis Medical Media, 1999: 149–156.

Shoskes DA, Zeitlin SI. Use of prostatic massage in combination with antibiotics in the treatment of chronic prostatitis. Prostate Cancer and Prostatic Diseases 1999; 2: 159–162.

Shoskes DA, Zeitlin SI, Shahed A, Rajfer J. Quercetin in men with category III chronic prostatitis: a preliminary prospective, double-blind, placebo control trial. Urology 1999; 34: 960–963.

Shurbaji MS, Gupta PK, Myers J. Immunohistochemical demonstration of chlamydial antigens in association with prostatitis. Mod Pathol 1998; 1: 348–351.

Simmons P, Thin R. Minocycline in chronic abacterial prostatitis: a double-blind prospective trial. Br J Urol 1985; 57: 43–45.

Siroky MB, Goldstein I, Krane RJ. Functional voiding disorders in men. J Urol 1981; 126: 200–204.

Smith JW, Jones SR, Reed WP et al. Recurrent urinary tract infections in men. Ann Intern Med 1979; 91: 544–548.

Stamey TA. Urinary tract infection in males. In: Stamey TA. Pathogenesis and treatment of urinary tract infections. Baltimore: Williams and Wilkins, 1980: 343–429.

Stamey TA, Meares EMJ, Winningham DG. Chronic bacterial prostatitis and the diffusion of drugs into prostatic fluid. J Urol 1970; 103: 187–194.

Stearns D. Seminal vesiculitis: a diagnostic problem. J Int Coll Surg 1963; 40: 354–363.

Stewart C. Prostatitis. Emerg Med Clin North Am 1988; 6: 391–402.

Sue DE, Chicola C, Brand-Zawadzki MN et al. MR imaging in seminal vesiculitis. J Comput Assist Tomogr 1989; 13: 662–664.

Sutor DJ, Wooley SE. The crystalline composition of prostatic calculi. Br J Urol 1974; 46: 533–535.

Suzuki T, Kurokawa K, Suzuki K, Matsumoto K, Yamanaka H. Transurethral balloon laser hyperthermia for chronic non-bacterial prostatitis: a clinical trial. Int J Urol 1995; 2: 29–32.

Szoke I, Torok L, D'Osa E et al. The possible role of anaerobic bacteria in chronic prostatitis. Int J Androl 1998; 21: 163–168.

Tan JK, Png DJ, Lieu LC et al. Prevalence of prostatitis-like symptoms (PS) in a population based study. J Urol 2001; 165 (Suppl 5): 23 (abstract 97).

Tanner MA, Shoskes DE, Shahed A, Pace NR. Prevalence of corynebacterial 16S rRNA sequences in patients with bacterial and "non-bacterial" prostatitis. J Clin Microbiol 1999; 37: 1863–1870.

Theodorou C, Konidaris D, Moutzouris G, Becopoulos T. The urodynamic profile of prostatodynia. BJU International 1999; 84: 461–463.

True LD, Berger RE, Rothman I, Ross SO, Kreiger JN. Prostate histopathology in chronic prostatitis/chronic pelvic pain syndrome, a prospective biopsy study. J Urol 1999; 162: 2014–2018.

VanHowe RS. Circumcision and infectious diseases revisited. Pediatr Infect Dis 1998; 17: 1–6.

Vassily O, Andrey S, Evgenii D et al. Efficacy of transrectal microwave hyperthermia (TRMH) in the treatment of chronic prostatitis. A randomized sham controlled comparative study. J Urol 1999; 161 (Suppl): 33A.

Veneziano S, Pavlica P, Mannini D. Color doppler ultrasonographic scanning in prostatitis: clinical correlation. Eur Urol 1995; 28: 6–9.

Vinje O, Fryjordet A, Bruu AL et al. Laboratory findings in chronic prostatitis – with special reference to immunological and microbiological aspects. Scand J Urol Nephrol 1983; 17: 291–297.

Von Lackum WH. Clinical and experimental data on prostatic infection. J Urol 1927; 18: 293–306.

Von Lackum WH. The infected prostate. Proc Staff Meetings Mayo Clinic 1928; 3: 14–16.

Wasserman Neil F. Prostatitis: clinical presentations and transrectal ultrasound findings. Semin Roentgenol 1999; 34: 325–337.

Webster GD, Lockhart JL, Older RA. The evaluation of bladder neck dysfunction. J Urol 1980; 123: 196–198.

Wedren H. Effects of sodium pentosanpolysulphate on symptoms related to chronic non-bacterial prostatitis. A double-blind randomized study. Scand J Urol Nephrol 1987; 21: 81–88.

Wedren H. On chronic prostatitis with special studies of Staphylococcus epidermidis. Scand J Urol Nephrol Suppl 1989; 123: 1–36.

Weidner W. Prostatitis – diagnostic criteria, classification of patients and recommendations for therapeutic trials. Infection 1992; 20: 227–231.

Weidner W, Ebner H. Cytological analysis of urine after prostatic massage (VB3): a new technique for discriminating diagnosis of prostatitis. In: Brunner H, Krause W, Rothaug CF, Weidner E (eds) Chronic Prostatitis. Stuttgart: Schattauer, 1985: 141–151.

Weidner W, Ludwig M. Diagnostic management of chronic prostatitis. In: Weidner W, Madsen PO, Schiefer HG (eds) Prostatitis – Etiopathology, Diagnosis and Therapy. Berlin: Springer, 1994: 158–174.

Weidner W, Brunner H, Krause W. Quantitative culture of *Ureaplasma urealyticum* in patients with chronic prostatitis or prostatosis. J Urol 1980; 124: 622–625.

Weidner W, Arens M, Krauss H, Schiefer HG, Ebner H. *Chlamydia trachomatis* in 'abacterial' prostatitis: microbiological, cytological and serological studies. Urol Int 1983; 38: 146–149.

Weidner W, Schiefer HG, Dalhoff A. Treatment of chronic bacterial prostatitis with ciprofloxacin. Results of a one-year follow-up study. Am J Med 1987; 82: 280–283.

Weidner W, Schiefer HG, Brahles E. Refractory chronic bacterial prostatitis: a reevaluation of ciprofloxacin treatment after a median followup of 30 months. J Urol 1991; 146: 350–352.

Weidner W, Schiefer HG, Krauss H, Jantos C, Friedrich HJ, Altmannsberger M. Chronic prostatitis: a thorough search for etiologically involved microorganisms in 1461 patients. Infection 1991; 19: 119–125.

Weinberger M, Cytron S, Servadio C et al. Prostatic abscess in the antibiotic era. Rev Infect Dis 1988; 10: 239–249.

Weiss JM. Pelvic floor myofascial trigger points: manual therapy for interstitial cystitis and the urgency-frequency syndrome. J Urol 2001; 166: 2226–2231.

Wenninger K, Heiman JR, Rothman I, Berghuis JP, Berger RE. Sickness impact of chronic nonbacterial prostatitis and its correlates. J Urol 1996; 155: 965–968.

Wishnow K, Wehner N, Stamey T. The diagnostic value of the immunologic response in bacterial and nonbacterial prostatitis. J Urol 1982; 127: 689–694.

Wright ET, Chmiel JS, Grayhack JT, Schaeffer AJ. Prostatic fluid inflammation in prostatitis. J Urol 1994; 152: 1–3.

Yamamoto M, Hibi H, Shatoshi A, Miyake K. Chronic bacterial prostatitis treated with intraprostatic injection of antibiotics. Scand J Urol Nephrol 1996; 30: 199–201.

Yavascaoglu I, Oktay B, Simsek U, Ozyurt M. Role of ejaculation in the treatment of chronic non-bacterial prostatitis. Int J Urol 1999; 6: 130–134.

Yoshimura T, Kurita C, Usami E et al. Immunomodulatory action of levofloxacin on cytokine production by human peripheral blood mononuclear cells. Chemotherapy 1996; 42: 459–464.

Young HH, Gereghty JT, Stevens AR. Chronic prostatitis. Johns Hopkins Hospital Rep 1906; 3: 271–384.

Zaichick VY, Sviridova TV, Zaichick SV. Zinc concentration in human prostatic fluid: normal, chronic prostatitis, adenoma and cancer. Int Urol Nephrol 1996; 28: 687–694.

Zerman DH, Ishigooka M, Doggweiler R, Schmidt RA. Chronic prostatitis: a myofascial pain syndrome? Infect Urol 1999; 12: 84–88.

Zermann DH, Schmidt RA. Neurophysiology of the pelvic floor: its role in prostate and pelvic pain. In: Nickel JC (ed) Textbook of Prostatitis. Oxford: Isis Medical Media, 1999: 95–105.

Zhang W, Sesterhenn IA, Connelly RR, Mostofi FK, Moul JW. Inflammatory infiltrate (prostatitis) in whole mounted radical prostatectomy specimens from black and white patients is not etiology for racial differences in prostate specific antigen. J Urol 2000; 163: 131–136.

Abbreviations: CPPS, chronic pelvic pain syndrome; LUT, lower urinary tract.

ALPHABETICAL INDEX

abacterial prostatitis,
     see non-bacterial prostatitis
abdominal ultrasound, 51
acute bacterial (category I) prostatitis,
     30, 32, 33, 56-7
   diagnosis, 32, 33, 39, 49
   presentation, 32
   treatment, 56-7
     algorithm, 82
α-adrenoceptor blockers,
     see alpha-blockers
alfuzosin in CPPS, 68
allopurinol, 74
alpha-blockers, 7
   chronic bacterial prostatitis, 60
   chronic pelvic pain syndrome, 68-9
amitriptyline, 74
anatomic abnormalities, 21
anesthesia and analgesia, *see* pain, relief
antiandrogens, 71
antibiotics, 7, 10-11
   acute bacterial prostatitis, 56
   asymptomatic inflammatory
     prostatitis, 79, 90-1
   chronic bacterial prostatitis, 58-60
   chronic pelvic pain syndrome, 65-6,
     86-7
     doses, 67
   era before, 10
anti-inflammatory agents, 7
   in CPPS, 69-70, 87-8
assessment (evaluation), 29-54, 83-4

asymptomatic inflammatory prostatitis
     (category IV prostatitis),
     31, 32, 79, 90-1
   PSA levels, 49
   treatment, 79, 90-1
autoimmune processes, 25

baclofen, 72
bacteria
   CPPS and, 66
   eradication, *see* antibiotics
   in etiology, 16-17, 18-19
     historical perspectives, 10-11, 16
     species implicated, 19
   evaluation, 29, 38, 39
     culture, *see* culture
   protective mode of survival in
     prostate, 18-19, 20, 66
bacterial prostatitis, 33, 56-61
   acute, *see* acute bacterial prostatitis
   chronic, *see* chronic bacterial
     prostatitis
   evaluation for/diagnosis of, 33, 38
   treatment, 56-61
bee pollen extract, 72, 73
biofeedback, 76
biofilms, bacterial, 19
bladder neck
   pathology (incl. obstruction),
     assessment, 22, 52, 53
   transurethral incision, 52, 78

cancer
   incidental diagnosis, 61
   urine cytology, 48

Alphabetical index continued

CAT scan, 51
categories, *see* classification
catheterization, urethral, 56
causation, *see* etiology
celebrex, 70
Chlamydia trachomatis, 17
chronic bacterial (category II) prostatitis,
    30-1, 32, 33, 58-61, 85-6
    diagnosis, 33, 39, 45
    presentation, 32, 33, 42
    treatment, 58-61
    algorithm, 85-6
chronic non-bacterial prostatitis,
    see chronic pelvic pain syndrome
chronic pelvic pain syndrome (category
    III prostatitis; prostatodynia and
    chronic non-bacterial prostatitis),
    31, 34, 62-78, 86-90
    diagnosis, 34, 40, 42, 45
    inflammatory, *see* inflammatory CPPS
    non-inflammatory,
        see non-inflammatory CPPS
    treatment, 62-78
    algorithm, 86-90
Chronic Prostatitis Symptom Index,
    NIH, 35-7
    CPPS treatment and, 62
classification (categories)
    NIH, 30-1, 32, 33-4
        diagnosis of specific categories,
            38-45, 47
        treatment of specific categories,
            56-79
    traditional, 12, 32
    see also specific categories

clinical presentation/features,
    see presentation; symptoms
clinical trials, *see* trials
computed tomography (CAT), 51
costs (economic), 3-4
co-trimoxazole, *see* trimethoprim
COX-2 inhibitors in CPPS, 69, 88
culture of bacteria, 29, 38, 39, 42, 45, 47
    mycoplasma, 47
cyclobenzaprine, 72
cyclooxygenase-2 inhibitors in CPPS, 69,
    82
cystitis
    interstitial, 26, 70
    previous history, 18
cystoscopy, 50
cytology, urine, 48

detrusor–bladder neck dyssynergia, 53
detrusor–sphincter dyssynergia, 53
diagnosis (of prostatitis), 7, 33-4, 94
    of different categories, 33-4
    differential, 46
    personnel involved, 6
    positive, percentage in primary care
        with, 6-7
diazepam, 72
diclofenac, 70
diet, 64
differential diagnosis, 46
doctors (physicians) in primary care, 6-9
doxazosin in CPPS, 68
drainage, urine, optimization, 56

drug therapy, 7-8
    acute bacterial prostatitis, 56
    asymptomatic inflammatory
        prostatitis, 79, 90-1
    chronic bacterial prostatitis, 58-60
    chronic pelvic pain syndrome, 65-74,
        86-8
    trials, 95
    see also specific (types of) drugs

economic costs, 3-4
electrical nerve stimulators, implantable,
    77
epidemiology, 2-3
etiology, 15-24, 94
    historical perspectives, 10-12, 16-17
    multifactorial factors, 26-7
evaluation, 29-54, 83-4
evidence-based management, 12, 93, 95

finasteride, 71, 82
fluoroquinolones, *see* quinolones
follow-up, acute bacterial prostatitis, 57
four-glass method, 12, 38, 39, 45, 83

gabapentin, 74
glycocalyx, bacterial, 19, 20, 66
gram-positive bacteria, 10, 16
    CPPS and, 66

heat therapy, local, 76-7
    self-administered, 64
histology, 11
historical perspectives, 10-13
    etiology, 10-12, 16-17

hormone therapy, 71
hyperthermia, transrectal, 77

ibuprofen, 70
imaging, 50-1
immunologic factors, 24, 26, 27
    see also autoimmune processes
incidence, 2-3
indomethacin, 70
infection, 10-11, 16-20
    historical perspectives, 10-11, 16-17
    previous history, 18-20
    see also bacterial prostatitis *and specific*
        microbes/pathogens
inflammation (in LUT), evaluation, 29
inflammatory CPPS (category IIIA
    prostatitis), 31, 32
    diagnosis, 40, 45, 47
    treatment algorithm, 87
inflammatory prostatitis, asymptomatic,
    see asymptomatic inflammatory
    prostatitis
injury, traumatic, 23-4, 26, 27
interstitial cystitis, 26, 70
investigations, *see* evaluation and specific
    methods

leukocytes (white blood cells) in prostatic
    secretions, 38, 40, 43, 44, 45
    in asymptomatic inflammatory
        prostatitis, 49
lifestyle changes, 64
lower urinary tract
    localization test, 38-45
    obstruction, *see* obstruction

Alphabetical index continued

magnetic resonance imaging (MRI), 51
malignancy, *see* cancer
massage, prostatic
    evaluating prostatic secretions/urine,
        38-40, 84
    technique, 41
    therapeutic use
        chronic bacterial prostatitis, 60
        chronic pelvic pain syndrome, 75
Meares-Stamey 4-glass method, 12, 38,
    39, 45, 84
microbiology, *see* infection *and specific*
    (types of) microbes
microscopy, 29
    prostatic secretions, 38, 43, 44
    semen, 47
    urine, 39
microwave thermotherapy, transurethral,
    77
micturition, *see* voiding
minimally invasive surgery, 76-7
MRI, 51
muscle relaxants, 71-2
Mycoplasma sp., 17-18
    culture, 47
myofascial trigger point release therapy,
    76

National Institutes of Health (NIH)
    Chronic Prostatitis Collaborative
        Research Network, 17
    Chronic Prostatitis Symptom Index,
        see Chronic Prostatitis
            Symptom Index
    classification by, *see* classification

nerve stimulators, implantable, 77
neurologic and neuromuscular
    mechanisms, 25, 26, 27
neuromodulation, 77
NIH, *see* National Institutes of Health
non-bacterial (abacterial) prostatitis
    chronic, *see* chronic pelvic pain
        syndrome
    evaluation for, 38
non-inflammatory CPPS (category IIIB
        prostatitis), 31, 32
    diagnosis, 40, 45
    treatment algorithm, 89
non-steroidal anti-inflammatory agents
        (incl. COX-2 inhibitors) in CPPS,
        69-70, 88

obstruction (to voiding/of LUT), 21
    urodynamic findings, 53
    voiding cystourethrogram, 22

pain (pelvic)
    location, 29
    relief (analgesia/anaesthesia), in
        CPPS, 88
        trigger point release therapy, 76
    see also chronic pelvic pain syndrome
pathogens, *see* infection *and specific (types*
    of) pathogen
pelvic neurologic system, 25, 27
pelvic pain, *see* chronic pelvic pain
    syndrome; pain
pelvic ultrasound, 51
pentosan sulfate, 70, 88

perineal trauma, 23-4, 26, 27

peripheral afferent nerve stimulation, 77

physical therapy, 75-6, 88-9

physicians (in primary care), 6-9

physiotherapy (physical therapy), 75-6, 88-9

phytotherapy, 72-3

plant extracts, 72-3

polymerase chain reaction, microbe detection, 18

presentation, 2, 29
    of different categories, 32
    see also symptoms

pressure–flow studies, 53

prevalence, 2-3

primary care physicians, 6-9

prostate
    anatomic abnormalities, 21
    cancer, *see* cancer
    massage, *see* massage
    protective mode of survival of bacteria in, 18-19, 20, 66
    secretions, evaluation, 38-40, 43, 44
    transurethral resection of (TURP), 78

prostate-specific antigen (PSA), 48-9
    asymptomatic inflammatory prostatitis and, 79, 90-1

prostatectomy, 78

Prostatitis Foundation, 95

prostatodynia, *see* chronic pelvic pain syndrome

PSA, *see* prostate-specific antigen

quality of life, 4-5

quercetin, 73

quinolones (incl. fluoroquinolones)
    chronic bacterial prostatitis, 58, 59
    chronic pelvic pain syndrome, 65, 86

radiology, 50-1

rectum, *see entries under* transrectal
    research, 95, 96
    see also trials

residual urine evaluation, 62

rofecoxib, 69, 70

sacral anterior nerve stimulation (SANS), 77

saw palmetto, 72, 73

semen analysis, 47

sexual dysfunction, 27, 29

Staphylococcus spp., 10, 16

Streptococcus spp., 10, 16

sulfamethoxazole–trimethoprim, *see* trimethoprim

supportive care, acute bacterial prostatitis, 57

surgery, 78
    bladder neck, 52, 78
    in chronic bacterial prostatitis, 60-1
    in CPPS, 78, 89-90
    minimally invasive, 76-7

swab, urethral, 47

symptoms
    assessment, 35-7
    bacteria as cause of, 17
    impact on quality of life, 4-5
    presenting, *see* presentation
    in treatment of CPPS, 62
    see also specific symptoms

Alphabetical index continued

tamsulosin in CPPS, 68, 69
terazosin in CPPS, 68
therapy, *see* treatment
thermotherapy, *see* heat therapy
transrectal hyperthermia, 77
transrectal ultrasound, 50-1
transurethral techniques, 76, 77, 78
    bladder neck incisions, 52, 78
trauma, 23-4, 26, 27
treatment, 55-92
    algorithms, 81-92
    future for, 95
    historical aspects, 10-11, 12
    ineffective, 27
    plans, 7-8, 55-80
trials, 95
    in CPPS, antibiotics, 66
trimethoprim (and trimethroprim–
        sulfamethoxazole
        [co-trimoxazole])
    chronic bacterial prostatitis, 58, 59
    chronic pelvic pain syndrome, 67
two-glass pre-/post-massage test,
        38-40, 45

ultrasound
    abdominal/pelvic, 51
    residual urine evaluation, 62
    transrectal, 50-1
Ureaplasma urealyticum, 17-18
urethra
    catheterization, 56
    swab, 47
    see also transurethral techniques

urethral sphincter–detrusor dyssynergia,
        53
urethritis, previous history, 18
urinary tract, lower, *see* lower urinary
        tract
urine
    drainage, optimization, 56
    residual, evaluation, 62
    specimens, evaluation, 38, 39
        cytological, 48
urodynamics, 52-3
uropathogenic bacteria, 16, 19
    evaluation for, 38, 39

videourodynamics, 52
voiding, obstruction, *see* obstruction
voiding cystourethrogram, bladder neck
        obstruction, 22

white blood cells, *see* leukocytes

zinc supplements, 73